Nursing Diagnosis and the Critically Ill Patient

Sharon L. Roberts, R.N., Ph.D.
Professor
Department of Nursing
California State University
Long Beach, California

Appleton
&Lange
Norwalk, Connecticut/Los Altos, California

Other books by Sharon L. Roberts:

Behavioral Concepts and the Critically Ill Patient, Second Edition

Physiological Concepts and the Critically Ill Patient

Copyright ©1987 by Appleton & Lange
A Publishing Division of Prentice-Hall

87 88 89 / 10 9 8 7 6 5 4 3 2 1

Prentice-Hall of Australia, Pty. Ltd., Sydney
Prentice-Hall Canada, Inc.
Prentice-Hall Hispanoamericana, S.A., Mexico
Prentice-Hall of India Private Limited, New Delhi
Prentice-Hall International (UK) Limited, London
Prentice-Hall of Japan, Inc., Tokyo
Prentice-Hall of Southeast Asia (Pte.) Ltd., Singapore
Whitehall Books Ltd., Wellington, New Zealand
Editora Prentice-Hall do Brasil Ltda., Rio de Janeiro

Library of Congress Cataloging-in-Publication Data

Roberts, Sharon L., 1942–
    Nursing diagnosis and the critically ill patient.
    1. Intensive care nursing. 2. Diagnosis. I. Title.
[DNLM: 1. Critical Care—nurses' instruction. 2. Nursing Assessment. WY 154 R647n]
RT120.I5R62 1987   616'.028   87-1500
ISBN 0-8385-7022-4

Design: Kathleen E. Peters

PRINTED IN THE UNITED STATES OF AMERICA

Contents

List of Abbreviations

ADH	Antidiuretic hormone
ADL	Activities of daily living
AMI	Acute myocardial infarction
APTT	Activated partial thromboplastin time
A–V	Atrial–ventricular
BEEP	Behavior, emotion, environment, and physiology
BND	Behavioral nursing diagnoses
bpm	Beats per minute
BUN	Blood urea nitrogen
CBC	Complete blood cell count
CHF	Congestive heart failure
CND	Collaborative nursing diagnoses
CNS	Central nervous system
CO	Cardiac output
CPAP	Continuous positive airway pressure
CPP	Cerebral perfusion pressure
CVA	Cerebrovascular accident
CVP	Central venous pressure
D&C	Dilation and curettage
DIC	Disseminated intravascular coagulation
DRGs	Diagnostic related groups
D/W	Dextrose/water
FANCAP	Fluid, aeration, nutrition, communication, activity, pain
GFR	Glomerular filtration rate
HLS	Hypertonic lactated saline
IABP	Intra-aortic balloon pump
ICP	Increased cardiac pressure

KVB	Kidney, ureter, bladder
LA	Left atrial
LOS	Length of stay
LVEDP	Left ventricular end diastolic pressure
MAP	Mean arterial pressure
MAST	Military anti-shock trousers
NANDA	North American Nursing Diagnosis Association
NDRGs	Nursing diagnostic related groups
NPO	Nothing by mouth
N/S	Normal saline
PA	Pulmonary artery
PAM	Mean pulmonary arterial pressure
PAC	Premature atrial contractions
PAP	Pulmonary artery pressure
PAT	Paroxysmal atrial tachycardia
PAW	Pulmonary artery wedge
PCWP	Pulmonary capillary wedge pressure
PEEP	Positive end expiratory pressure
PJB	Premature junctional beat
PMI	Point of maximum intensity (impulse)
PT	Prothrombin time
PTT	Partial thromboplastin time
PVB	Premature ventricular beat
PVR	Pulmonary vascular resistance
S-A	Sinoatrial
SAP	Systemic artery pressure
SBP	Systemic blood pressure
SIADH	Syndrome of inappropriate anti-diuretic hormone
SVP	Systemic venous pressure
SVR	Systemic vascular resistance
TIA	Transient ischemic attacks
URI	Upper respiratory infection
UTI	Urinary tract infection
V½P	Ventilation perfusion
VT	Ventricular tachycardia
WBC	White blood cell count

1

Introduction

Nursing is a dynamic profession requiring change and subsequent management of a growing complexity of patient problems or needs. This dynamic quality has long been experienced by nurses working in the fast-paced and often highly-technical area known as *critical care*. Nurses in this area are confronted with a multitude of patient problems and needs. In many instances, it is the critical care nurse who identifies potential problems and relates pertinent data to a physician.

Nurses have always been actively involved in identifying specific patient problems. Now nurses are incorporating these problems into a new framework referred to as *nursing diagnosis*. In response to the growing need for the creation of a classification system whereby nurses can utilize their own terminology regarding nursing diagnosis, the National Conference Group for Classification of Nursing Diagnosis was organized in 1973. The group has since been renamed the North American Nursing Diagnosis Association (NANDA). NANDA's purpose is to facilitate the acceptance of a common list of nursing diagnosis and to clarify the meaning of the term itself (Kelly, 1985). The group is to be commended for its efforts in developing a list of acceptable nursing diagnoses.

One of the current problems with nursing diagnosis is the lack of understanding or under use of those diagnoses that have been accepted by NANDA and by the profession in general. While the currently accepted nursing diagnosis list has merit and application for the nurse generalist, it lacks the same applicability for critical care nurses. The reason for this is a lack of physiologically related nursing diagnoses. The lack of such diagnoses is particularly significant for critical care nurses who are confronted with numerous physiological problems each day. According to Tanner: "Attempts to limit the nursing diagnoses used in practice to only those appearing on the accepted list are likely to result in frustration, confusion, and incomplete documentation of care provided" (1985, p. 424).

There are times when the physiological needs of clients are the greatest with behavioral needs becoming more evident as physiological stability is achieved. In addition, the few acceptable physiological nursing diagnoses, such as fluid-volume excess or deficit, are very general. The diagnoses need to be further specified into intracellular and extracellular fluid-volume excess or deficit. It has taken critical care nurses and clinical specialists more than twenty years to develop the specificity of their knowledge base. Therefore, there is a growing need for a way to incorporate the critical care nurse's knowledge base into what is called *collaborative nursing practice*. According to Kim, "collaboration in nursing is conceptually related both to the manner of professional practice and the client–professional relationship (1983, p. 272). It also applies to the professional relationship between nurse and physician.

There is yet another reason for increasing the number of behavioral and physiological nursing diagnoses: reimbursement. Recently, President Reagan signed Public Law 98-21, the Social Security Amendment of 1983. Title VI of this law changes the way that Medicare determines how much hospitals are reimbursed for inpatient care. The prospective payment system, based on Diagnostic-Related Groups (DRGs), bring clinical and financial data together. Reimbursement is based upon the particular DRG assigned to a Medicare patient (Shaffer, 1984). Similar changes may take place within nursing practice. Instead of DRGs, reimbursement for nursing care received may be based upon Nursing Diagnostic-Related Groups (NDRGs).

PURPOSE OF THE TEXT

In the past, nursing practice has been based upon a dependent relationship with the medical profession. Nurse clinicians have provided direct patient care based upon a biomedical model built upon medical diagnosis. Today, clinicians and academicians recognize that nurses are capable of performing their skills interdependently or collaboratively with, and independently from, the traditional biomedical model. Critical care nurses can increase their skill and knowledge in diagnostic judgment with continued practice in diagnostic thinking. Like physicians, nurses collect data regarding a patient's potential or actual health problem; analyze the data by isolating significant findings; cluster related facts and attach meaning to the clusters; and, finally, state a nursing diagnosis (Kelly, 1985). Therefore, the movement for independence in nursing practice is being achieved through the development of theory and nursing science.

Collaboration implies sharing information. This signifies that each participant in the health care system respects the other's knowledge level. Nursing care of the critically ill patient is enhanced when integrated together with the contributions of other health professionals. Collaboration also requires that nurses and physicians rethink their clinical decision making in an attempt to recognize the contributions of each to patient care. As nurses become proficient in formulating both collaborative and behavioral nursing diagnoses, autonomy will increase. Nurses will realize a sense of value in the care that they provide.

The nursing diagnosis movement has gained a popularity during the past several years that is relatively new to the majority of nurses. There is still disagreement over what constitutes a nursing diagnosis and how it should be applied to various areas of practice, such as critical care. The current use of nursing diagnoses implies that nurses must describe nursing problems or needs that fall within the jurisdiction of independent nursing practice. Tanner points out two points of disagreement: "(1) the extent to which nursing diagnosis taxonomy should attempt to describe the entire scope of nursing practice, encompassing health problems that nurses treat independently with other disciplines, and (2) whether physiological nursing diagnoses should be excluded from the taxonomy because their treatment usually requires medical collaboration" (1985, p. 424).

Gordon advocates the use of nursing diagnoses to describe only independent nursing practice. For Gordon, many of the physiological diagnoses (alteration in cardiac output and fluid-volume deficit/excess) require referral to a physician or treatment following medical protocol, thereby failing to meet the criteria for a nursing diagnosis (1979). Likewise, Tanner notes that Carnevali subscribes to the belief that critical care nurses must assume a high degree of responsibility in the biomedical domain, but this is not the domain of nursing diagnosis (1985). Guzetta and Dosey believe that nurses' dependent and independent roles do not exist in critical care nursing practice and that most of the critical care nurse's role is interdependent (1983, p. 281).

Kim (1984), on the other hand, is a proponent of physiological and/or collaborative nursing diagnoses. She believes that physiological diagnoses are clinically relevant to nurses and are well within the scope of nursing practice. Tanner summarizes three key factors supporting Kim's position. First, while nursing is typically viewed as health-oriented, ill persons hospitalized with altered physiological functioning will continue to need the attention of the nursing profession. Second, physiological diagnoses do not represent the renaming of medical diagnoses and are not the exclusive domain of medicine. Third, the boundaries between nursing and medicine are not so distinct that independent nursing practice can be clearly defined (1985).

Kim's belief in the relevance of physiological nursing diagnoses gives credence to the need for further development of collaborative or physiological nursing diagnosis. For clinicians and academicians involved in critical care nursing, there is a growing need for physiological nursing diagnosis as it pertains to medical diagnosis or DRGs. Collaborative nursing diagnoses focus on the physiological needs of the patient. Collaboration necessitates both medical and nursing interventions in order to restore the individual to a level of wellness. In this respect, both disciplines work together. A nurse may have a collaborative diagnosis of "cardiac pressure, alteration in: increased left ventricular–atrial preload"; "decreased cardiac output"; or, "cardiac rhythm, alteration in: sinus tachycardia." With each of these physiological or collaborative diagnoses, the contribution of both medicine and nursing to the therapeutic plan of a critically ill patient is recognized. The diagnoses do require both nursing and medical interventions. In this respect, nursing integrates with medicine but, in doing so, it does not lose its separate identity.

In addition, it seems appropriate to develop subcategories under generally accepted nursing diagnoses. For example, the nursing diagnosis "tissue perfusion, alteration in" can be further delineated into collaborative subnursing diagnoses, listed as follows:

Tissue Perfusion, Alteration in
Collaborative Subnursing Diagnoses
Coronary artery perfusion decreased
Peripheral tissue perfusion decreased
Peripheral tissue perfusion obstructed: thrombophlebitis
Vasodilatation of vascular bed: anaphylactic shock
Pulmonary tissue perfusion alteration: emboli
Cerebral perfusion obstructed: thromboembolism
Vasodilatation of vascular bed: neurogenic shock
Renal tissue perfusion decreased

It appears that this diagnostic category would be more useful to nurses working in coronary care, respiratory care, neurological care, and hemodialysis if the subcategories were developed as subnursing diagnoses. For example, a hemodialysis nurse might be concerned about his or her patient's renal tissue perfusion in relationship to a hypotensive crisis or postanesthetic reaction. Therefore, the hemodialysis nurse might diagnose "renal tissue perfusion decreased" within the larger diagnostic category of "tissue perfusion, alteration in."

Hence, the purpose of this textbook is to (1) apply existing nursing diagnoses to critical care; (2) further specify certain nursing diagnoses; and (3) develop additional behavioral/psychological and physiological nursing diagnoses. For the purpose of this text, psychosocial nursing diagnoses are referred to as behavioral nursing diagnoses (BND) in order to separate them from physiologically-based nursing diagnoses, referred to as collaborative nursing diagnoses (CND). For example, a critical care nurse may assess regulatory and cognitive behaviors (defining characteristics), evaluate arterial blood gasses, auscultate the chest, and evaluate the data from hemodynamic parameters before diagnosing a patient's problem as ventilation-perfusion imbalance. The nurse's actions in arriving at the diagnosis are independent. The nurse then collaborates with the patient's physician, who confirms the diagnosis and follows prescribed treatments. The nurse will follow prescribed treatments as well as carry out independent nursing responsibilities, some of which are delineated under the diagnosis of ventilation-perfusion imbalance. The nursing diagnosis *ventilation-perfusion imbalance* is important and reflects the nurse's use of physical assessment skills and his or her sophisticated knowledge base. Therefore, collaborative diagnoses need to be developed and used by nurses working in the dynamic and highly specialized area of critical care. Nursing interventions will be suggested, with each intervention designated as dependent (D), interdependent (ID), or independent (I).

DEFINITIONS

Nursing diagnoses can be differentiated into behavioral or collaborative nursing diagnoses. Psychosocial nursing diagnoses are referred to as behavioral nursing diagnoses, whereas physiologically based nursing diagnoses are collaborative diagnoses. According to Kim: "Collaboration is defined as a process in which two or more individuals work together for the attainment of a goal; a process by which a joint influence on an action is produced" (1983, p. 276).

> *Behavioral Nursing Diagnosis:* A cluster of signs and symptoms describing an actual or potential health problem that nurses, because of their education and expertise, are licensed and able to treat (Gordon, 1976, p. 1298).

> *Collaborative Nursing Diagnosis:* A cluster of signs and symptoms describing an actual or potential health problem such that the nurse consults or collaborates with a physician in order to arrive at the appropriate treatment.

According to Kim: "The level of collaboration may be conceptualized as a continuum on which the lowest collaboration is expressed as complete domination of decision making by the nurse and the highest level of collaboration is expressed as an equally influencing joint decision making" (1983, p. 280).

Defining characteristics or signs and symptoms can be further broken down into regulatory and cognitive behaviors. In this respect, a nurse may assess both types of behaviors, each of which may present themselves at different times during the patient's hospitalization in critical care.

> *Regulatory Behaviors:* Regulatory behaviors are physiological responses.

> *Cognitive Behaviors:* Cognitive behaviors are behavioral/psychological responses.

Finally, nursing responsibilities can be divided into two components; namely, assessment and intervention. Each intervention is categorized according to whether or not it is independent, interdependent, or dependent.

> *Independent Intervention:* An intervention that does not require a physician's order.

> *Interdependent Intervention:* An intervention that requires consultation with a physician and expert judgment by the nurse.

> *Dependent Intervention:* An intervention that requires a physician's order and that may involve the administration of drugs or specific invasive treatment and may require the use of protocols or standing orders.

OVERALL FRAMEWORKS

The overall framework consists of three parts. First, the nursing diagnoses are organized around the assessment tool BEEP—Behavior, Emotion, Environment, and Physiology. Psychological and physical assessment are significant components of the nursing process and are utilized by nurses working in various critical care units. Furthermore, the critical care nurse draws upon knowledge of physical assessment skills to assist in the formulation of a nursing diagnosis for an individual suffering from physical dysfunction.

Today, critical care nurses make observations and judgments about their patients. Nurses have become more knowledgable in the contributing science and more competent in analytical thinking, so that they are able to make decisions and diagnoses without waiting for medical direction. Critical care nurses are filled with vital information designed to correlate with alterations in the patient's physiological status. Prepared with knowledge about how to care for the critically ill patient at his or her bedside, the nurse can produce valuable information and can supply specific actions designed either to assist the patient in recovering from illness or to provide supportive care in a pleasant manner. The nurse has the responsibility of assessing, intervening, evaluating, and diagnosing, while simultaneously maintaining a caring relationship with each of his or her patients.

The BEEP concept helps the nurse to make quick and thorough assessments of any critically ill patient and to formulate a nursing diagnosis that may be correlated with the medical-domain diagnosis for critical care patients. When a nurse approaches a patient, he or she must have a starting point determined by the nature and severity of the patient's illness. BEEP enables the nurse to begin at any of the four major levels, helping him or her to organize assessments into categories and to conclude with an overall nursing diagnosis. The concept provides a logical, sequential method of making observations for each major level (Roberts, 1986).

A patient's behavior can be indicative of potential physiological problems or needs. The patient who complains of tiredness or lethargy may in fact be hypokalemic or anemic. Behaviors may range from cognitive responses (such as restlessness, lethargy, aggressiveness, or confusion) to regulatory behaviors (such as tachycardia, hypertension, or dyspnea). The behavioral component of BEEP consists of patient consciousness, behavior consistency, the characteristics of a patient's background, and his or her movement control.

Emotional assessment, the second component, involves assessing the emotional factors confronting a patient as he or she copes with an illness, injury, or trauma. An individual's emotional reaction may be confined to one response, (such as anger), or a cluster of responses, (such as denial, powerlessness, or anxiety). The emotional component enables the nurse to look beyond surface behaviors to their emotional origin. For example, the patient's behavior may change from jovial to withdrawn. The nurse may diagnose the change in behavior as denial. Emotional assessment deals with components such as feelings of loneliness, frustration, hopelessness, powerlessness, anger, depression, fear of loss, alteration in self-concept, separation, failure to be personalized and to accept denial, and frustration due to pain.

Environmental assessment is the examination of the patient's immediate environment for factors contributing to his or her behavioral emotional response. Admission into a critical care unit, with its sophisticated instrumentation, may be a new and frightening experience to the patient. The continuous bombardment of strange stimuli may lead to behaviors of paranoia, confusion, combativeness, or hallucination. The nurse assesses the patient's behavior and evaluates the presence of excessive environmental stimuli coupled with sleep deficit to arrive at the nursing diagnoses of sleep deprivation and sensory overload. In this case, the environmental components include stimuli from the environment, sensory overload, sensory deprivation, sleep deprivation, and stress.

The physiological component is an assessment tool designed to direct the nurse's data-collection process from head (sclera color) to toe (status of major system). Physiological components include sclera color; status of pupils; skin color; status of central venous pressure; status of pulmonary pressures; systolic and diastolic pressure; sounds in chest, heart, and bowel; and status of cardiovascular, pulmonary, renal, neurological, gastrointestinal, and endocrine systems. Only the status of the six systems will be utilized in the physiological section.*

Next, nursing responsibilities are presented according to assessment and interventions that have been organized around the nursing care model of FANCAP. In reviewing current discussions of interventions within the nursing diagnosis framework, nurses are including assessment and are observing and monitoring actions as interventions. These are not interven-

---

*For a detailed discussion of the assessment tool BEEP, refer to *Behavioral Concepts and the Critically Ill Patient*, 2nd ed. by Sharon L. Roberts. Norwalk, Conn.: Appleton-Century-Crofts, 1986.

tions but, rather, data-collecting tools. Therefore, for each behavioral or collaborative nursing diagnosis presented, the nursing responsibilities covered will be divided into their assessment and intervention components.

The nursing care model, FANCAP, consists of the following: fluid, aeration, nutrition, communication, activity, and pain (Abbey, 1980). Fluid can mean any liquid or solution taken in or put out by a patient. Fluid can also signify pressure, volume resistance, viscosity, flux, gradients, concentrations, forces, compartments, and spaces. Aeration implies the movement or exchange by which oxygen is made available to the lungs and tissues and by which the metabolic gaseous and products are eliminated. The lungs are aerated through ventilation, making certain that the airway is patent, the thorax moves, and sufficient quantities of oxygen are available for inhalation. In addition, ventilation also implies opening up so that the individual can ventilate or discuss their problems. Aeration pertains to providing oxygen to the lungs or tissues and to the psychological ventilation of a problem. The third component, nutrition, goes beyond the obvious nourishment of the patient; the concept pervades all related disciplines and cultures. In this respect, nutrition can encompass psychological nutrition, cognitive nutrition, cultural nutrition, and spiritual nutrition. Communication signifies that the patient is conveying a message or thought through verbal and/or nonverbal means. It also implies an exchange or feedback between the patient and factors within the environment and family. For example, the nurse assesses whether lines, wires, or tubes are open or communicating with the patient. Thus, all treatments or supportive devices are observed to see if they are providing the necessary exchange or feedback with the patient. Activity is multifocal, involving physical, mental, cardiac, endocrine, and renal activity. Pain consists of physiological pain attributed to injury, stretching, or a lack of oxygen and of psychological pain attributed to fear, loneliness, hopelessness, or anxiety.*

---

*For a further discussion of FANCAP, refer to *Physiological Concepts and the Critically Ill Patient* by Sharon L. Roberts. Englewood Cliffs, N.J.: Prentice-Hall, 1985.

Carpenito, L. J. *Handbook of nursing diagnosis*. Philadelphia: Lippincott, 1984.

DeGasperis, M. Implementing nursing diagnosis in the critical care setting. *Dimensions of Critical Care Nursing*, 2(1), January–February 1983.

Gettrust, K., Ryan, S. & Engleman, D. *Applied nursing diagnosis*. New York: Wiley, 1985.

Gordon, M. *Manual of nursing diagnosis*. New York: McGraw-Hill, 1985.

Guzetta, C. E. and Dossey, B. M. Nursing diagnosis: Framework, process and problems. *Heart & Lung*, 12, 281, 1983.

Kelly, M. A. *Nursing diagnosis source book*. Norwalk, Conn.: Appleton-Century-Crofts, 1985.

Kim, M. J. Nursing diagnosis in critical care. *Dimensions of Critical Care Nursing*, 2(1), January–February 1983.

Kim, M. J., McFarland, G., & McLane, A. *Nursing diagnosis*. St. Louis: C. V. Mosby, 1984.

Kim, H. S. Collaborative decision making in nursing practice: A theoretical framework. In P. Chinn (ed.), *Advances in nursing theory development*. Rockville, Md.: Aspen Systems Corporation, 1983.

Lengel, N. *Handbook of nursing diagnosis*. Bowie, Md.: Robert J. Brady, 1982.

Roberts, S. *Behavioral concepts and the critically Ill patient* (2nd ed.). Norwalk, Conn.: Appleton-Century-Crofts, 1986.

Roy, C. and Roberts, S. *Theory construction in nursing*. Englewood Cliffs, N.J.: Prentice-Hall, 1981.

Tanner, C. Symposium on nursing diagnosis in critical care. *Heart & Lung*, 14(5), 423–425, September 1985.

Shaffer, F. A. A nursing perspective of the DRG world: Part 1, *Nursing & Health Care*, 5, 48–51, 1984.

Gordon, M. The concept of nursing diagnosis, *Nursing Clinics of North America*, 14, 487–496, 1979.

Gordon, M. Nursing diagnosis and the diagnostic process, *American Journal of Nursing*, 76, 1298–1300, 1976.

2

Diagnostic Category List

---

*New behavioral/social or physiological nursing diagnosis.
†Nursing diagnosis on the accepted list.
CND = collaborative nursing diagnosis; BND = behavioral nursing diagnosis.

*New behavioral/social or physiological nursing diagnosis.
†Nursing diagnosis on the accepted list.
 CND = collaborative nursing diagnosis; BND = behavioral nursing diagnosis.

*New behavioral/social or physiological nursing diagnosis.
†Nursing diagnosis on the accepted list.
  CND = collaborative nursing diagnosis; BND = behavioral nursing diagnosis.

Note: Those nursing diagnoses on the accepted list but not included in text: Home maintenance management altered; Health maintenance altered; Parenting, alteration in; Social isolation; Social interaction, impaired; Rape trauma syndrome.

*New behavioral/social or physiological nursing diagnosis.

†Nursing diagnosis on the accepted list.

  CND = collaborative nursing diagnosis; BND = behavioral nursing diagnosis.

3

Behavioral Assessment

The critical care nurse makes observations and assessments regarding consciousness, consistency of behavior, characteristics of patient background, and control of movement. By quickly assessing these components, the nurse obtains baseline information for making judgments about a patient's care or progress. If the nurse observes a deviation, he or she can begin gathering additional data in an attempt to formulate the nursing diagnosis and appropriate intervention.

CONSCIOUSNESS OF PATIENT

The patient will be responsive or unresponsive, oriented or disoriented, communicative or noncommunicative.

THOUGHT PROCESS ALTERED, CONFUSION

DEFINITION
Confusion arises from pathology involving circulation, oxygenation, and metabolism of the brain leading to inattention and memory deficits, inappropriate verbalizations, disruptive behavior, noncompliance, and failure to perform activities of daily living.

ETIOLOGY
Hypoxia
    Blood loss
    Iron deficiency
    Pernicious anemia

Hypothermia
Hyperthermia
Dehydration
Electrolyte imbalance
Hypocalcemia
Alzheimer
Uremia
Congestive heart failure
Increasing intracranial pressure
Hypothyroidism
Hypotension
Hypoxemia
Emphysema
Pneumoconiosis
Byssinosis
Glucose excess or deficiency
Hyperglycemia
Hypoglycemia
Drug effect
Digitalis toxicity
Alcohol excess
Sedatives, tranquilizers, and narcotics
Stress
Visual deficits
Blindness
Diplopia
Hearing deficits
Total loss of hearing
Tinnitus
Tactile deficits
Diminished ability to sense touch

DEFINING CHARACTERISTICS
Regulatory Behaviors
Tachycardia
Elevated blood pressure
Arrhythmias
Diaphoresis
Incontinence
Cognitive Behaviors
Disorientation

Impaired attention span
Restlessness
Anxiety
Apprehension
Fear
Agitation
Incoherent speech
Withdrawal
Belligerence
Combativeness
Delusions
Depression
Impaired memory
Difficulty concentrating
Unable to recognize others

NURSING RESPONSIBILITIES

Assessment

Assess regulatory behaviors indicative of confusion (I)
Assess cognitive behaviors indicative of confusion (I)
Monitor the ECG pattern continuously (I)
Observe the side or therapeutic effects of prescribed medications (I)
Assess the patient's level of consciousness (I)
Assess prehospital episodes of confusion (I)
Monitor situations or factors contributing to confusion (I)
Auscultate the heart for abnormal heart sounds (I)
Auscultate the heart for rate, rhythm, and regularity (I)
Palpate the pulses for quality and bilateral equality (I)
Inspect the skin color, temperature, and presence of diaphoresis (I)
Inspect for dehydration (I)
Inspect the jugular veins for distension (I)
Auscultate the chest for adventitious breath sounds (I)
Auscultate the chest for respiratory rate, rhythm, and regularity (I)
Inspect for cyanosis (I)
Inspect for dyspnea (I)
Palpate the chest for vocal or tactile fremitus (I)
Percuss the chest for abnormal resonance (I)

Interventions

Fluids
   Administer prescribed IV fluids (D)
   Administer prescribed medications (D)
   Regulate the IV flow rate and check for patency (I)
   Measure intake, output, and specific gravity (I)
   Evaluate laboratory studies: serum electrolyte, hemoglobin, hematocrit, blood urea nitrogen (BUN), and creatine (I)
   Evaluate data from hemodynamic parameters: pulmonary artery pressure (PAP), pulmonary capillary wedge pressure (PCWP), central venous pressure (CVP), systemic vascular resistance (SVR), and cardiac output (CO) (I)
   Measure arterial blood pressure and mean arterial pressure (MAP) (I)

Aeration
   Administer humidified oxygen via mask, nasal catheter, or nasal prongs at the prescribed flow rate (D)
   Establish and maintain a patent airway (I)
   Evaluate arterial blood gasses (I)
   Reduce meaningless environmental stimuli (I)

Nutrition
   Assist the patient with diet (I)
   Provide the patient with the prescribed diet (I)
   Adjust the diet to the person's lifestyle (I)
   Provide a spiritual support system (I)

Communication
   Ask questions that encourage answers that reflect reality perception (I)
   Keep teaching on a simple level (I)
   Protect the patient from injury while confused (I)
   Listen to the patient's confused behavior and assist with reality orientation (I)
   Listen to the family concerns, fears, and anxieties (I)
   Reduce the patient's anxiety level (I)
   Reassure the patient that the confusion is temporary (I)
   Reduce the demand for cognitive functioning when the person is ill or fatigued (I)

Activity

    Change the patient's position q2h (I)
    Encourage alternative rest and supervised activity (I)
    Encourage diversional activity (I)
    Orient the patient to time, place, and location (I)
    Encourage patient interactions with family and staff (I)

Pain

    Administer prescribed analgesics (D)
    Evaluate the type, location, and duration of the pain (I)
    Reassure the patient that the pain will subside or be relieved (I)
    Ask the patient what makes him or her comfortable (I)

Bibliography

Carpenito, L. J. *Handbook of nursing diagnosis.* Philadelphia: Lippincott, 1984.

Gettrust, K., Ryan, S., & Engleman, D. *Applied nursing diagnosis.* New York: Wiley, 1985.

Kim, M. J., McFarland, G., & McLane, A. *Nursing diagnosis.* St. Louis: C. V. Mosby, 1984.

Wolanin, M. & Phillips, L. *Confusion prevention and care.* St. Louis: C. V. Mosby, 1981.

COMMUNICATION, IMPAIRED VERBAL
Verbal/Nonverbal Communication Deficit

DEFINITION

A state in which the individual experiences reduced or absent verbal/nonverbal communication.

ETIOLOGY

    Alteration in thought process
    Ineffective listening skills
    Cerebral impairment
        Central nervous system (CNS) depression
        Tumor
        Trauma
        Hypoxia

Neurological impairment
   Quadriplegia
   Myasthenia gravis
   Multiple sclerosis
Auditory impairment
Respiratory impairment
   Shortness of breath
Laryngeal edema
Language barrier
Memory deficit
Trauma to face, mouth, or hands
Speech pathology
Endotracheal intubation
Tracheostomy
Drugs
Fear

DEFINING CHARACTERISTICS

Regulatory Behaviors
Muscle tension
Shortness of breath
Decreased auditory comprehension
Deafness

Cognitive Behaviors
Withdrawal
Silence
Does not finish sentence
Lack of eye contact
Refusal to speak
Short attention span
Weak or absent voice
Confusion

NURSING RESPONSIBILITIES

Assessment
Assess regulatory behaviors indicative of communication deficit (I)
Assess cognitive behaviors indicative of communication deficit (I)

Assess the patient's prehospital communication pattern (I)
Assess situations or factors contributing to communication deficit (I)
Inspect the patient for dyspnea or shortness of breath (I)

Intervention

Fluid

Administer prescribed medications (D)
Evaluate the patient for physiological reasons as to the communication deficit (I)

Aeration

Provide the patient with a pen and clipboard and help patient to verbalize in written form (I)
Create an environment conducive to verbal participation (I)
Reduce meaningless environmental stimuli (I)
Provide a quiet environment with a distraction of the patient's choice, such as radio or television (I)

Nutrition

Provide prescribed diet (I)
Assist the patient with eating (I)

Communication

Encourage the patient to verbally participate in his or her care and with staff (I)
Listen to the patient when he or she communicates (I)
Provide alternative means of communication for those patients temporarily unable to communicate (I)
Insert a hearing aid (I)
Reduce the patient's anxiety level (I)
Encourage communication between the patient and family (I)
Encourage patient participation in self-care (I)
Provide support and encouragement when the patient does verbally respond (I)
Evaluate the type of communication deficit disorder (I)
Speak with the patient when in the patient's room (I)
Explain all procedures (I)

Activity

Encourage moderate physical activity (I)

Change the dependent patient's position q2h (I)

Reduce the demand for cognitive functioning when the patient is ill or fatigued (I)

Encourage patient participation in diversional activity (I)

Encourage the patient's family and friends to visit and communicate with the patient (I)

Pain

Evaluate the type, location, and duration of pain (I)

Evaluate for nonverbal cues of pain, such as facial grimaces, clutched fists, increased pulse, increased blood pressure, and diaphoresis (I)

Administer prescribed medications (D)

Ask the patient what makes him or her comfortable (I)

Bibliography

Gettrust, K., Ryan, S., & Engleman, D. *Applied nursing diagnosis.* New York: Wiley, 1985.

Verbal/Nonverbal Communication Excess

DEFINITION

A state in which the individual experiences excessive verbal/nonverbal communication output.

ETIOLOGY

Alcohol intake

Drugs

Trauma

Mental disorders

Congestive heart failure

Hypoxemia

Chronic renal failure

Hepatic failure

Burn trauma

Fear

Anxiety

DEFINING CHARACTERISTICS

Regulatory Behaviors

Tachycardia

Elevated blood pressure
Diaphoresis

Cognitive Behaviors
Rapid speech
Incoherent speech
Exaggeration
Aggressive behavior
Argumentativeness
Loose association
Defensive
Inappropriate speech
Anxiousness

NURSING RESPONSIBILITIES

Assessment
Assess regulatory behaviors indicative of communication excess (I)
Assess cognitive behaviors indicative of communication excess (I)
Assess the patient's prehospital communication pattern (I)
Assess situations or factors leading to communication excess (I)
Inspect the respiration for rate, rhythm, and regularity (I)

Intervention

Fluid
Administer prescribed medications (D)
Evaluate the patient for physiological reasons as to the communication excess (I)

Aeration
Create a relaxed environment conducive to anxiety reduction (I)
Create an environment in which patient can verbalize his or her feelings in a nonaggressive manner (I)

Nutrition
Provide the prescribed diet (D)
Assist the patient with eating (I)

Communication
Reduce the patient's anxiety level (I)

Listen to the patient's concerns and frustrations (I)

Calmly communicate with the patient in an attempt to reduce his or her aggressive behavior (I)

Realize that excess communication behavior is a symptom
of other problems (I)

Encourage decision making (I)

Evaluate the type of communication excess disorder (I)

Explore with the patient reasons for self-criticism or
negativism (I)

Explore with the patient previous achievements or successes
(I)

Consult with both physician and psychologists (I)

Activity

Reduce purposeless or combative physical activity (I)

Help the patient to channel excess energy into diversional
activities or meaningful communication (I)

Reduce the demand for cognitive functioning when the
patient is ill or fatigued (I)

Prepare the patient for all nursing interventions (I)

Pain

Administer prescribed analgesics (D)

Evaluate for the presence or absence of pain (I)

Ask the patient what makes him or her comfortable (I)

Bibliography

Gettrust, K., Ryan, S., & Engleman, D. *Applied nursing diagnosis.* New
York: Wiley, 1985.

CONSISTENCY OF BEHAVIOR

The critical care nurse may assess inappropriate or sudden
changes in behavior, such as sudden withdrawal from environmental interaction and noncompliance with treatment
modalities. A once-quiet patient may suddenly become violent.
The patient may direct his or her violence toward him- or
herself or toward others within the environment.

NONCOMPLIANCE

DEFINITION
A state in which the individual's informed decision is not to adhere to a therapeutic recommendation, such as exercise, medication, or follow-up care.

ETIOLOGY
Denial of illness, injury, or disease
Depression
Fatigue
Health beliefs
Cultural beliefs
Lack of knowledge
Lack of perceived benefits of therapeutic intervention
Lack of significant others
Pain
Loss of control
Inability to perform tasks
Financial concerns
Lack of autonomy
Inability to make decisions
Poor self-esteem
Alteration in body image

DEFINING CHARACTERISTICS

Regulatory Behaviors
Complications
Exacerbations of symptoms
Altered laboratory tests
Decreased muscle strength
Inability to perform exercises

Cognitive Behaviors
Verbalization of noncompliance
Partially used or unused medications
Failure to keep appointments
Failure to progress
Withdrawal
Failure to seek care when needed

NURSING RESPONSIBILITIES

Assessment

Assess regulatory behaviors indicative of noncompliance (I)

Assess cognitive behaviors indicative of noncompliance (I)

Assess prehospital noncompliance with medication, diet, appointments, or exercise (I)

Interventions

Fluid

Administer prescribed medications (D)

Evaluate whether or not the patient is taking prescribed medications (I)

Evaluate laboratory studies that indicate whether or not the patient is complying with the therapeutic regime (I)

Aeration

Reduce meaningless environmental stimuli (I)

Create a supportive environment conducive to compliance (I)

Nutrition

Determine the patient's food preferences and provide favorite foods within dietary restrictions (ID)

Assist the patient with eating (I)

Encourage the patient to comply with the prescribed diet (I)

Review the dietary intake with the patient to determine adherence to the prescribed diet (I)

Adjust the diet to the patient's lifestyle (I)

Communication

Listen to the patient's reasons for noncompliance (I)

Involve the patient in an exercise program (I)

Teach the patient the importance of complying with dietary restrictions (I)

Provide knowledge regarding illness and therapeutic measures (I)

Involve both patient and family in planning follow-up care (I)

Emphasize the positive aspects of follow-up care (I)

Encourage patient self-performance (I)

Emphasize the importance of adhering to dietary restrictions when the patient is discharged (I)

Teach the patient the importance of adhering to his or her medication regimen (I)

Determine the patient's knowledge level regarding his or her drug therapy and instruct when the patient's knowledge seems insufficient (I)

Inform the patient regarding the action of medications that he or she is to use at home, when realistic (I)

Advise the patient to consult with a physician before taking any medications that might be incompatible with prescribed medications (I)

Inform the patient to notify his or her physician of any side effects while taking medication (I)

Encourage the patient to ventilate his or her concerns regarding drug therapy (I)

Activity

Encourage family members to participate in the patient's activity program (I)

Encourage alternative rest and activity periods (I)

Encourage the use of passive/active range-of-motion exercises (I)

Pain

Administer analgesics as prescribed (D)

Evaluate the type, location, and duration of pain (I)

Determine if pain is the reason for noncompliance (I)

Bibliography

Carpenito, L. J. *Handbook of nursing diagnosis.* Philadelphia: Lippincott, 1984.

Gettrust, K., Ryan, S., & Engleman, D. *Applied nursing diagnosis.* New York: Wiley, 1985.

Kim, M. J., McFarland, G., & McLane, A. *Nursing diagnosis.* St. Louis: C. V. Mosby, 1984.

VIOLENCE DIRECTED TOWARD SELF

DEFINITION

A state in which the individual experiences violent, aggressive, and self-destructive acts or feelings.

ETIOLOGY
  Temporal lobe epilepsy
  Loneliness
  Alcohol
      Intoxication
      Sudden withdrawal
  Drug abuse
  Toxic reaction to medication
  Neurological impairment
      Organic brain syndrome
      Cerebral tumor
  Hormonal imbalance
  Manic depression
  Rage reaction
  Stressor
  Prolonged physical immobility
  Suicidal behavior
  Fear of the unknown
  Loss of significant others

DEFINING CHARACTERISTICS

Regulatory Behaviors
  Increased motor activity
  Rigid body language
  Tachycardia

Cognitive Behaviors
  Fear
  Anxiety
  Delusion
  Hallucination
  Agitation
  Depression
  Perception of self as worthless or hopeless
  Psychotic thought process
  Threat of personal loss

NURSING RESPONSIBILITIES

Assessment
  Assess regulatory behaviors indicative of violence directed
      toward self (I)

Assess cognitive behaviors indicative of violence directed toward self (I)

Assess prehospital factors contributing to self-directed violence (I)

Monitor situations or factors causing the patient to direct violence toward self (I)

Interventions

Fluid

Administer prescribed medications to control agitated behaviors (D)

Evaluate the symptoms of self-directed behavior and determine their severity (I)

Evaluate the patient's environment for harmful items (I)

Aeration

Create a relaxed environment (I)

Reduce stressful events in the immediate environment (I)

Nutrition

Assist the patient with his or her diet (I)

Adjust the diet to the patient's lifestyle (I)

Incorporate the patient's cultural preferences into diet when possible (I)

Communication

Establish basic trust and rapport with the patient (I)

Listen to the patient's concerns, fears, and anxieties (I)

Approach the patient in a positive supportive manner (I)

Establish limits if the patient is unable to do so (I)

Reduce the patient's outside responsibilities (I)

Reduce anxiety-producing interactions with others (I)

Reinforce reasons to live (I)

Assist the patient in identifying strengths (I)

Encourage patient self-performance (I)

Encourage the patient to strive toward realistic goals (I)

Encourage patient acceptance of self-limitations (I)

Reinforce use of positive problem-solving skills (I)

Encourage the patient to express feelings and clarify situation (I)

Activity

Seclude and/or restrain the patient if he or she is unable to control own behavior (I)

Limit purposeless physical activity (I)
Encourage involvement of significant other(s) (I)
Supervise independent physical activity (I)

Pain
Evaluate the type, location, and duration of pain (I)
Administer prescribed analgesics (D)

Bibliography

Carpenito, L. J. *Handbook of nursing diagnosis.* Philadelphia: Lippincott, 1984.
Gettrust, K., Ryan, S., & Engleman, D. *Applied nursing diagnosis.* New York, Wiley, 1985.
Kim, M. J., McFarland, G., & McLane, A. *Nursing diagnosis.* St. Louis: C. V. Mosby, 1984.

VIOLENCE DIRECTED TOWARD OTHERS

DEFINITION
A state in which the individual experiences violent, aggressive, and destructive acts or feelings directed toward others in the environment.

ETIOLOGY
Physical trauma
Alcohol
Intoxication
Sudden withdrawal
Drug abuse
Feeling of alienation
Psychotic thought process
Social isolation
Threat of personal loss
Perceived threat to self-esteem
Misperceived messages from others
Antisocial character
Rage reactions

DEFINING CHARACTERISTICS

Regulatory Behaviors
Tachycardia
Increased motor activity

Cognitive Behaviors

Hostile threats or rage directed toward others
Combativeness
Overt aggressive acts directed toward others
Suspicion of others
Perception of the environment as frightening or hostile

NURSING RESPONSIBILITIES

Assessment

Assess regulatory behaviors indicative of violence directed toward others (I)
Assess cognitive behaviors indicative of violence directed toward others (I)
Assess prehospital experiences of violence directed toward others (I)
Assess situations or factors contributing to violence directed toward others (I)

Interventions

Fluid

Administer prescribed medications to control agitated behaviors (D)
Evaluate the symptoms of other-directed violence and determine its severity (I)
Evaluate the patient's environment for harmful items (I)

Aeration

Create a safe, relaxed environment (I)
Reduce stressful events in the immediate environment (I)
Reduce meaningless environmental stimuli (I)

Nutrition

Assist the patient with his or her diet (I)
Adjust the diet to the patient's lifestyle (I)

Communication

Evaluate the patient's effective coping devices and strategies (I)
Listen to the patient's concerns and fears (I)
Determine the meaning behind the patient's violent behavior (I)
Help the patient to identify the reasons for his or her behavior (I)

Reinforce the use of positive coping strategies (I)
Reduce the number of people who interact with the patient
(I)

Activity
Restrain the physically aggressive patient (I)
Limit purposeless physical activity (I)
Encourage meaningful interaction with others (I)

Pain
Evaluate the type, location, and duration of pain (I)
Administer prescribed analgesics (I)
Ask the patient what makes him or her comfortable (I)

Bibliography

Carpenito, L. J. *Handbook of nursing diagnosis.* Philadelphia: Lippin-
cott, 1984.
Gettrust, K., Ryan, S., & Engleman, D. *Applied nursing diagnosis.* New
York: Wiley, 1985.
Kim, M. J., McFarland, G., & McLane, A. *Nursing diagnosis.* St. Louis:
C. V. Mosby, 1984

CHARACTERISTICS OF PATIENT BACKGROUND

The most important characteristic of the critically ill patient's
background is an overall patient history. Other characteristics
to be determined are personal idiosyncrasies about the patient,
including his or her occupation, education level, marital status,
number of children, hobbies, roles assumed, sexuality, and
family structure.

DIVERSIONAL ACTIVITY DEFICIT

DEFINITION
When the individual's environment is devoid of meaningful or
purposeful stimuli or the individual is unable to structure time
to avoid boredom.

ETIOLOGY
Environment devoid of diversional activity
Supportive devices or intrusive procedures limiting diver-
sional activity

ETIOLOGY

Illness of a family member
Fear of death
Separation from the sick family member
Sudden onset of illness without warning
Unfamiliarity of the critical care environment
Unfamiliarity of the critical care team
Potential financial crisis
Lack of knowledge regarding illness, diagnostic procedures, and prognosis
Unfamiliarity with supportive devices connected to a family member
Personal external stressors (e.g., small children, job)
Role conflict
Incongruent values, goals, or beliefs
Unrealistic future goals
Personality conflict within the family
Interpersonal conflict with the sick family member
Loneliness
Hopelessness

DEFINING CHARACTERISTICS

Regulatory Behaviors
Not applicable

Cognitive Behaviors
Helplessness
Decreased problem-solving ability
Fear
Anxiety
Panic
Withdrawal
Crying
Apathy
Inability to meet physical, social, emotional, or spiritual needs of family members
Inability to seek or accept outside help
Unrealistic expectations
Altered sleep pattern

Anger
Despair
Overprotectiveness toward the sick family member
Withdrawal
Role confusion
Manipulation of others
Shortened attention span
Disorganized thought process
Expression of guilt or blaming
Argumentative behavior
Agitation

NURSING RESPONSIBILITIES

Assessment

Assess the family unit's pre-crisis coping strategies (I)
Monitor situations contributing to the crisis within the family unit (I)
Observe cognitive behaviors indicative of a family crisis (I)
Assess the family's readiness for learning (I)

Interventions

Fluid

Provide individualized and supportive care by identifying and acknowledging the family's needs (I)
Provide feedback regarding data obtained from diagnostic procedures (I)
Explain the purpose behind supportive devices used in critical care (I)

Aeration

Encourage the use of a spiritual support system (I)

Nutrition

Evaluate the family's nutritional status since the illness of a family member (I)

Communication

Provide the family with information by answering and reanswering their questions (I)
Assist the family in identifying alternative coping behaviors (I)

Foster communication between the family and the sick family member (I)

Provide flexible visiting hours (I)

Listen to the family's verbalization of concerns, fears, and anxieties (I)

Instruct the family as to the nature of the illness, diagnostic procedures, and progress (I).

Help the family to accept potential role changes (I)

Provide information regarding community resources (I)

Encourage the family to make realistic future goals (I)

Assist the family in making decisions for the sick family member (I)

Encourage the family to participate in the patient's care, when realistic (I)

Activity

Prepare the family for what they will see in critical care (I)

Encourage the family to participate in group education sessions with families experiencing similar situations (e.g., cardiac bypass) (I)

Pain

Not applicable

Bibliography

Beard, M. The impact of hemodialysis and transplantation on the family. *Critical Care Quarterly*, 1, 87–91, September 1978.

Beosworth, J. & Molen, M. Psychological stress in spouses of patients with myocardial infarction. *Heart and Lung*, 11(5), 450–456, September–October 1982.

Carpenito, L. J. *Handbook of nursing diagnosis*, Philadelphia: Lippincott, 1984.

Dunkel, J. & Eisendroth, S. F. Families in the intensive care unit: Their effect on staff. *Heart and Lung*, 12, 258, 1983.

Gettrust, K., Ryan, S., & Engleman, D. *Applied nursing diagnosis.* New York: Wiley, 1985.

Gordon, M. *Manual of nursing diagnosis.* New York: McGraw-Hill, 1985.

Kim, M. J., McFarland, G., & McLane, A. *Nursing diagnosis.* St. Louis: C. V. Mosby, 1984.

Roberts, S. *Family in crisis: Behavioral concepts and the critically ill patient* (2nd ed.). Norwalk, Conn.: Appleton-Century-Crofts, 1986.

KNOWLEDGE DEFICIT

DEFINITION
The individual experiences a deficiency in cognitive knowledge.

ETIOLOGY
    Lack of understanding
    Language difficulty
    Lack of recall
    Cultural differences
    Medications
    Lack of motivation
    Complexity of information
    Denial of situation
    Anxiety
    Depression
    Lack of interest
    Information misinterpretation
    Cognitive limitations

DEFINING CHARACTERISTICS

Regulatory Behaviors
    Unknown

Cognitive Behaviors
    Verbalizes lack of knowledge
    Noncompliance
    Inaccurately uses the information given
    Hysteria
    Agitation
    Apathy
    Requests information
    Misconception

NURSING RESPONSIBILITIES

Assessment
    Assess regulatory behaviors indicative of knowledge deficit
        (I)
    Assess cognitive behaviors indicative of knowledge deficit (I)
    Assess the patient's understanding of his or her illness and
        treatments associated with his or her disease (I)

Interventions

Fluid

Teach the patient about hemodynamic parameters, need for invasive procedures, and medications (I)

Aeration

Teach the patient about the need for oxygen and/or ventilatory support (I)

Reduce extraneous environmental stimuli (I)

Nutrition

Assist the patient with eating (I)

Communication

Instruct the patient regarding the causes of his or her particular problem (I)

Listen to the patient's concerns (I)

Establish an individualized teaching program that takes into account the patient's cognitive ability (I)

Reduce the patient's anxiety level (I)

Encourage the patient to ask questions (I)

Consult with the patient's physician to determine any unique treatment modalities that will be used with the patient (I)

Teach the patient in a quiet environment free from interruptions (I)

Provide material in small increments so as not to overload the patient (I)

Ask the patient questions in order to determine whether or not he or she understands the material (I)

Review the material that the patient does not understand or recall (I)

Encourage the patient when learning does occur (I)

Encourage the patient's family to participate in the learning process (I)

Involve other patients who have the same diagnosis to participate in the teaching program (I)

Provide learning material that the patient can take home after his or her discharge (I)

Activity

Encourage physical activity to motivate the patient (I)

Provide diversional activity (I)

Pain
   Evaluate the type, location, and duration of pain (I)
   Administer prescribed analgesics (D)

Bibliography

Carpenito, L. J. *Handbook of nursing diagnosis.* Philadelphia: Lippin-
   cott, 1984.
Kim, M. J., McFarland, G., & McLane, A. *Nursing diagnosis.* St. Louis:
   C. V. Mosby, 1984

ROLE DISTURBANCE

DEFINITION
A perceived or actual state in which the individual is unable to
perform role obligations or expectations.

ETIOLOGY
   Alteration in physiological status
   Financial loss
   Prolonged hospitalization
   Alteration in family structure
   Change in employment
   Loss of employment
   Ineffective coping mechanism
   Loss of role
   Lack of support group
   Role conflict
   Low self-concept

DEFINING CHARACTERISTICS
Regulatory Behaviors
   Physical impairment
   Reduced capacity to perform role

Cognitive Behaviors
   Change in self-perception of role
   Denial
   Lack of knowledge
   Difficulty performing the role
   Stated inability to perform role expectations
   Anger

NURSING RESPONSIBILITIES

Assessment

Assess regulatory behaviors indicative of role disturbance (I)

Assess cognitive behaviors indicative of role disturbance (I)

Assess prehospital factors contributing to role disturbance (I)

Assess coping strategies used in handling role disturbance (I)

Assess situations or factors in critical care contributing to role disturbance (I)

Intervention

Fluid

Evaluate physiological reasons for role disturbance (I)

Aeration

Reduce environmental stimuli threatening role performance (I)

Create an environment conducive for role performance (I)

Nutrition

Provide the prescribed diet (I)

Assist the patient with eating (I)

Communication

Listen to the patient's concerns regarding role change (I)

Encourage both patient and family to discuss possible role changes (I)

Reduce the patient's anxiety regarding the consequences of role changes (I)

Anticipate and provide for the patient's needs (I)

Arrange situations that encourage the patient's autonomy (I)

Encourage patient self-performance (I)

Encourage patient acceptance of self-limitations (I)

Explore with the patient previous achievements or successes (I)

Activity

Encourage physical activity (I)

Encourage the patient to participate in the planning of future goals (I)

Pain
   Administer prescribed medications (D)
   Ask the patient what relieves his or her discomfort (I)

SEXUAL DYSFUNCTION

DEFINITION
A potential or actual condition in which the individual experiences a change in sexual health or sexual function different from the usual adequate or rewarding pattern.

ETIOLOGY
   Diabetes mellitus
   Hyperthyroidism
   Addison's disease
   Acromegaly
   Myxedema
   Chronic renal failure
   Arthritis
   Multiple sclerosis
   Neuromuscular disorder
   Myocardial infarction
   Congestive heart failure
   Chronic obstructive pulmonary disease
   Cancer
   Liver disease
   Fear
   Fatigue
   Anxiety
   Pain
   Depression
   Lack of knowledge
   Medications
   Low self-concept
   Altered body image
   Alcohol
   Radiation treatment
   Absence of sexual teaching
   Ileostomy
   Colostomy

DEFINING CHARACTERISTICS

Regulatory Behaviors
    Weakness on one side of the body
    Spasticity
    Hyperactive tendon reflexes
    Babinski's sign
    Facial weakness

Cognitive Behaviors
    Anxiety
    Fear
    Nervousness
    Confusion

NURSING RESPONSIBILITIES

Assessment
    Assess regulatory behaviors indicative of hemiparesis (I)
    Assess cognitive behaviors indicative of hemiparesis (I)
    Monitor the ECG pattern continuously (I)
    Observe the side or therapeutic effects of prescribed medi-
        cations (I)
    Assess the patient's neurological status: pupillary reaction,
        sensory–motor changes, level of consciousness, and vital
        signs (I)
    Auscultate the heart for rate, rhythm, and regularity (I)
    Auscultate the chest for respiratory rate, rhythm, and regu-
        larity (I)
    Auscultate the chest for normal and abnormal breath
        sounds (I)

Intervention

Fluid
    Administer appropriate IV fluids (D)
    Administer prescribed medications (D)
    Regulate the IV flow rate and check for patency (I)
    Measure arterial blood pressure and MAP (I)
    Measure intake and output (I)
    Evaluate laboratory studies (I)

Aeration

Suction the patient as ordered and as required (prn) (D)
Administer oxygen at the prescribed flow rate (D)
Evaluate for dyspnea (I)
Maintain a patent airway (I)

Nutrition

Assist the patient with diet (I)
Include the patient's favorite foods, if possible (I)
Evaluate the patient's ability to chew and swallow (I)

Communication

Evaluate the patient's communication pattern (I)
Inform the physician of changes in the patient's condition (I)
Reduce the patient's anxiety level (I)
Listen to the patient's concerns (I)
Encourage the patient to strive toward realistic goals (I)

Activity

Reposition and turn the dependent patient q2h (I)
Assist the patient in moving in bed (I)
Evaluate for abnormal physical activity or movement (I)

Pain

Administer prescribed medications (D)
Evaluate the type, location, and duration of pain (I)
Evaluate the patient's perception of and/or sensitivity to pain (I)
Reassure the patient that the pain will subside or be relieved (I)

Bibliography

Hickey, J. *Clinical practice of neurological and neurosurgical nursing.* Philadelphia: Lippincott, 1981.
Rutkowski-Conway Long, B. *Neurological and neurosurgical nursing.* St. Louis: C. V. Mosby, 1982.

Impaired Physical Mobility, Hemiplegia

DEFINITION

Hemiplegia is defined as paralysis of one side of the body.

Evaluate for the presence of cough, gag, and swallow reflexes (I)

Evaluate arterial blood gasses (I)

Nutrition

Provide the prescribed diet (D)

Adjust the diet to the patient's lifestyle (D)

Assist the patient with eating (I)

Evaluate the presence and quality of chewing ability (I)

Evaluate the presence and quality of swallowing (I)

Communication

Reduce the patient's anxiety level (I)

Listen to the patient's concerns and fears (I)

Provide spiritual support for family members or significant others (I)

Anticipate and provide for the patient's needs (I)

Keep teaching on a simple-to-complex level, depending upon the patient's level of understanding (I)

Provide knowledge regarding the causes of the patient's weakness (I)

Inform the physician of any changes in respiratory status (I)

Activity

Evaluate the muscular strength of all groups with repetitive activity (ID)

Protect the patient from injury (I)

Evaluate the patient's speech quality and ability (I)

Encourage alternative rest and supervised activity periods (I)

Evaluate for abnormal body movement (I)

Change the patient's position q2h (I)

Pain

Administer prescribed analgesics (D)

Evaluate the type, location, and duration of pain (I)

Bibliography

Johanson, B., Dungca, C., Hoffmeister, D., & Wells, S. *Standards for critical care* (2nd ed.). St. Louis: C. V. Mosby, 1985.

Sumi, S. M., Ruff, R., & Swanson, P. *Motor disturbance: Signs and symptoms in neurology.* Philadelphia: Lippincott, 1984.

Wyngaarden, J. & Smith, L. *Cecil textbook of medicine.* Philadelphia: Lippincott, 1984.

PSYCHOLOGICAL IMMOBILITY

DEFINITION
Immobility reduces the quality and quantity of sensory information available to the individual and reduces the ability of the individual to interact with his or her environment.

ETIOLOGY
Environmental factors
> Supportive services
> Loss of familiar belongings
> Stressors, such as noise or lights
> Unfamiliar critical care team

Illness
> Loss of bodily part
> Trauma
> Anxiety
> Loss of biological function

Role disturbance
> Estrangement from family or significant others
> Alteration in self-image
> Lifestyle changes
> Self-conflict
> Loss of social activities
> Dependence
> Financial concerns

DEFINING CHARACTERISTICS

Regulatory Behaviors
Fatigue
Anorexia
Loss of weight
Numbness of body part

Cognitive Behaviors
Withdrawal
Depression
Anger
Lassitude
Apathy
Memory disturbance

Nursing Responsibilities

Assessment

Assess the existence of prehospital psychological immobility (I)

Assess situations contributing to psychological immobility (I)

Assess the significance that illness has for the patient (I)

Interventions

Fluid

Explain and remove extraneous supportive devices (I)

Aeration

Minimize unfamiliar environmental noises (I)

Create a familiar environment (I)

Nutrition

Incorporate the patient's lifestyle and preferences into the diet, when possible (I)

Communication

Provide family contact (I)

Instruct the patient regarding the biological implications of his or her illness or injury (I)

Listen to the patient's expression of anxiety, frustration, and perception-impression of a threat to his or her existence (I)

Help the patient to find meaning in his or her illness (I)

Provide an atmosphere that encourages a positive self-concept (I)

Encourage the patient to use his or her illness experience in developing a more enduring sense of identity (I)

Activity

Provide diversional activities to move away from the patient's focus on the sick organ (I)

Encourage physical mobility (I)

Pain

Discuss with the patient measures to reduce his or her pain (I)

Evaluate whether or not pain is the cause of psychological immobility (I)

Bibliography

Roberts, S. *Psychological immobility: Behavioral concepts and the critically ill patient* (2nd ed.). Norwalk, Conn.: Appleton-Century-Crofts, 1986.

Roberts, S. Psychological equilibrium. In M. Kinney, C. Dean, D. Packa, & D. Voorman (eds.) *AACNs clinical reference for critical care nursing.* New York: McGraw-Hill, 1981, pp. 331–341.

Illness
Denial
Anger
Depression
Anxiety
Feelings of isolation
Analgesics
Physical immobilization
Sleep deprivation

DEFINING CHARACTERISTICS

Regulatory Behaviors
Numbness of body part
Inability to move
Increased heart rate
Increased respiratory rate
Fatigue
Loss of appetite
Dizziness
Flatness of visual and auditory stimuli

Cognitive Behaviors
Obsessional thinking
Low self-esteem
Doubt
Insecurity
Depression
Anxiety
Giddiness
Uselessness
Loss of affective responsiveness
Remoteness
Feeling of being dead

NURSING RESPONSIBILITIES

Assessment
Assess situations in which feelings of depersonalization occur (I)

Monitor statements reflecting a sense of depersonalization (I)

Intervention

Fluid

Explain the purpose behind supportive devices and the need for technological surveillance (I)

Personalize nursing care (I)

Aeration

Provide meaningful touch (I)

Nutrition

Incorporate the patient's food preferences into his or her diet, when possible (I)

Encourage a family member or significant other to eat with the patient (I)

Communication

Treat the critical care patient as a unique individual (I)

Explain the relationship between biological illness and diagnostic or treatment procedures (I)

Instruct the patient regarding biological illness and progress (I)

Provide feedback regarding the effectiveness of treatment modalities (I)

Encourage family participation (I)

Establish a personal communication link with both patient and family (I)

Activity

Motivate the patient to participate in care and to make decisions (I)

Pain

Administer prescribed analgesics (D)

Evaluate the type, location, and duration of pain (I)

Bibliography

Kleck, H. ICU syndrome: Onset, manifestations, treatment, stressors and prevention. *Critical Care Quarterly*, 6(4), 21–28, March 1984.

Levy, J. & Wachtel, P. Depersonalization: An effort at clarification. *American Journal of Psychoanalysis*, 38, 291–300, 1978.

Roberts, S. *Depersonalization: Behavioral concepts and the critically ill patient* (2nd ed.). Norwalk, Conn.: Appleton-Century-Crofts, 1986, pp. 276–297.

Torch, E. M. Review of the relationship between obsession and deper-
    sonalization. *ACTA Psychiatric Scand*, 58, 191–198, 1978.

FEELINGS OF POWERLESSNESS

Powerlessness can be assessed first as loss of control involving
physiological loss of control, psychological loss of control,
and environmental loss of control. Secondly, powerlessness
can be as a lack of knowledge.

POWERLESSNESS

DEFINITION
The expectation or belief held by the individual that his or her
own behavior cannot determine the outcome of reinforcements
that he or she seeks (Seeman, 1959).

OTHER DEFINITIONS

Alienation
A complex, impairing process whereby an individual experiences a loss of awareness and a blurring of the inner emotions
as a result of the sum total of his or her life experiences
(Yoder, 1977).

Power
The potential or actual ability of an individual to influence,
cause, or prevent changes in the cognition, attitude, behavior,
or emotions of another individual in interpersonal relation-
ships.

ETIOLOGY
    Loss of control
        Physiological
        Psychological
        Environmental
    Lack of knowledge
    Lack of motivation

DEFINING CHARACTERISTICS

Regulatory Behaviors
   Tiredness
   Fatigue
   Dizziness
   Headache
   Gastrointestinal disturbance

Cognitive Behaviors
   Apathy
   Withdrawal
   Resignation
   Fatalism
   Malleability
   Low knowledge of illness
   Statements of low control
   Anxiety
   Restlessness
   Sleeplessness
   Wandering
   Aimlessness
   Lack of decision making
   Aggression
   Anger

NURSING RESPONSIBILITIES

Assessment
   Assess situations in which the patient feels powerlessness (I)
   Monitor ways in which the critical care nurse inadvertently
      creates feelings of powerlessness in patient (I)

Interventions

Fluid
   Inform the patient when his or her biological problems have
      stabilized (I)
   Provide knowledge regarding the temporary limitations of
      illness and its complications (I)

Aeration
   Provide environmental control by allowing the patient to

decide where he or she would like personal belongings placed (I)

Nutrition

Encourage the patient to participate in decisions pertaining to his or her diet (I)

Communication

Encourage the patient to identify situations in which he or she feels powerless (I)

Restore control by removing the discrepancy between the patient's condition and his or her ideal self (I)

Provide the patient with a feeling of security regarding his or her own biological well-being (I)

Restore control by encouraging the patient to express concerns, fears, and anxieties (I)

Encourage the patient to establish realistic goals (I)

Listen to the patient's discussion regarding possible role changes and financial concerns (I)

Activity

Help the patient to regain control through decision making (I)

Pain

Identify whether or not pain is causing a feeling of powerlessness (I)

Bibliography

Miller, J. F. Development and validation of a diagnostic label: powerlessness in Kim, M. J., McFarland, G. & McLane, A. (eds.), *Classification of nursing diagnosis: proceedings of the fifth national conference.* St. Louis: C. V. Mosby, 1984.

Roberts, S. *Powerlessness: Behavioral concepts and the critically ill patient* (2nd ed.). Norwalk, Conn.: Appleton-Century-Crofts, 1986, 173–196.

Seeman, M. On the meaning of alienation. *American Sociological Review*, 24, 783–791, December 1959.

Wilkinson, M. Power and the identified patient. *Perspective in Psychiatric Care*, 17(6), 248–253, 1979.

Yoder, S. Alienation as a way of life. *Perspective in Psychiatric Care*, 15(2), 66–71, 1977.

FEELINGS OF ANGER

There are two general characteristics of anger and hostility expression to be assessed: the perception of a threat and the location of the agent of harm. The critically ill patient's display of anger may be the only energy output or control system that he or she feels is possible in a strange, unyielding environment.

ANGER

DEFINITION
A conflictive emotion that, on the biological level, is related to aggressive systems and, even more important, is related to the capacities for cooperative social living, symbolization, and reflective self-awareness. On the psychological level, anger is aimed at the correction of some appraised wrong; on the sociocultural level, it functions to uphold accepted standards of conduct (Averill, 1982, p. 317).

ETIOLOGY
    Anger expression inhibited: Internalization
        Perceived threat
            Blocked goal
            Failure of individuals to live up to the patient's expectations
            Disappointment
            Blow to self-view
            Illness perceived to be life-threatening
            Physical dependence
            Altered social integrity
        Agent of harm located
            Authoritative figure (staff) perceived to be threatening
            Family
            Self
    Anger directly expressed: Externalization
        Perceived threat
            Obstructed goal
            Role changes
            Financial dependence

Agent of harm located
Environment
Critical care team

DEFINING CHARACTERISTICS

Regulatory Behaviors
Increased blood pressure
Increased pulse rate
Increased respiration
Muscle tension
Perspiration
Flushed skin
Nausea
Dry mouth

Cognitive Behaviors
Clenched muscles or fists
Turned-away body
Avoidance of eye contact
Tardiness
Silence
Sarcasm
Insulting remarks
Verbal abuse
Argumentativeness
Demanding

NURSING RESPONSIBILITIES

Assessment
Assess prehospital situations contributing to expressions of anger (I)
Monitor behavior leading to internalization or externalization of anger (I)
Observe family interactions that might contribute to expressions of anger (I)
Assess regulatory behaviors indicative of anger (I)
Assess cognitive behaviors indicative of anger (I)

Interventions

Fluid

Help the patient to identify positive aspects of his or her illness (I)

Aeration

Accept the patient's behavior without judgment (I)

Nutrition

Encourage the patient to participate in decisions regarding his or her diet (I)

Communication

Provide a line of communication whereby the patient can express angry feelings (I)

Help the patient to identify situations in which he or she feels anger (I)

Explore the reasons behind angry feelings (I)

Explain ways in which the patient's behavior can change (I)

Activity

Assist the patient in finding alternate ways of coping with loss of control, powerlessness, or dependence (I)

Pain

Evaluate whether or not pain is causing feelings of anger (I)

Bibliography

Averill, J. *Anger and aggression: An essay on emotion.* New York: Springer-Verlag, 1982.

Knowles, R. Handling anger: Responding vs. reaching. *American Journal of Nursing*, 81(2), 2196, December 1981.

Roberts, S. *Hostility and anger: Behavioral concepts and the critically ill patient*, (2nd ed.). Norwalk, Conn.: Appleton-Century-Crofts, 1986, pp. 144–172.

FAILURE TO ACCEPT: DENIAL

Denial can be assessed according to direct-action tendencies, which consist of actions aimed at eliminating or reducing potential harmful events (threats). The events can be categorized according to those directly expressed (avoidance with fear), fear with avoidance (expression inhibited), or avoidance without fear. Secondly, denial is assessed according to defense reappraisal, whereby denial is used to reduce anxiety by minimizing the individual's perception of the threat (Roberts, 1986).

DENIAL

DEFINITION
A defense mechanism operating outside of any conscious awareness in the endeavor to resolve emotional conflict and so allay anxiety (Kiening, 1978). Goldberger (1983) has identified three types of denial: major, partial, and minimal. Major denial describes patients who state that they have experienced no fear at any time throughout their hospitalization or at any time earlier in their lives. Partial denial describes the patient who initially denies being frightened but eventually admits experiencing some fear. Minimal denial applies to patients who complain of anxiety or admit to feeling frightened.

ETIOLOGY
Potential limitations of illness
Hospitalization
Environment
Threat of role changes
Financial concerns
Physical restrictions
Lack of decision-making power
Stress
Dependence
Unrealistic perceptions
Vulnerability and potential death

DEFINING CHARACTERISTICS

Regulatory Behaviors
Tachycardia
Tachypnea
Normal or increased blood pressure
Angina
Arrhythmias

Increased urinary catecholamines
Gastrointestinal discomfort

Cognitive Behaviors
Rationalization
Displacement
Magical thinking
Isolation
Tunnel vision
Selective perception
Withdrawal

NURSING RESPONSIBILITIES

Assessment
Assess regulatory behaviors indicative of denial (I)
Assess cognitive behaviors indicative of denial (I)
Assess prehospital situations in which denial was used (I)
Monitor statements made by the patient reflecting denial of
his or her illness outcome (I)
Assess circumstances in which the patient uses denial (I)

Intervention

Fluid
Administer prescribed medications (D)
Explain the purpose behind supportive devices (I)

Aeration
Listen to the patient's reasons for denial in confronting a
perceived threat or harmful agent (I)

Nutrition
Encourage the patient to eat the prescribed diet (I)
Encourage a family member or significant other to eat with
the patient (I)

Communication
Provide knowledge regarding illness and complications as
they pertain to the individual patient (I)
Help the patient to accept his or her illness, or disfigurement (I)

NURSING RESPONSIBILITIES

Assessment

Assess regulatory behaviors indicative of self-concept/self-esteem disturbance (I)

Assess cognitive behaviors indicative of self-concept/self-esteem disturbance (I)

Assess prehospital events fostering a positive self-concept/self-esteem (I)

Assess prehospital self-esteem (I)

Monitor hospital events leading to self-concept/self-esteem disturbance (I)

Interventions

Fluid

Assist the patient in identifying positive aspects of illness (such as surviving the crisis, becoming closer to loved ones, etc.) (I)

Aeration

Provide supportive atmosphere designed to foster positive self-concept (I)

Nutrition

Include patient in decisions regarding his or her diet, when possible (I)

Communication

Help the patient to identify alternative coping behaviors (I)

Provide knowledge regarding illness, trauma, or disease (I)

Encourage family support and involvement (I)

Encourage the patient to develop realistic future goals (I)

Assist the patient in making realistic expectations of him- or herself (I)

Listen to the patient's expression of inadequacies (I)

Evaluate with the patient roles that will not change within the family unit, workplace, social activities, and hobbies (I)

Encourage the patient to verbalize his or her feelings (I)

Assist the patient in identifying new activities or modifications in old, familiar activities that will support a positive self-concept (I)

Encourage the patient's family to allow the patient to continue to perform family, work, and home responsibilities permitted by the limitations of his or her illness or treatment (I)

Identify with the patient possible maladaptive coping mechanisms that alter his or her self-concept and, through listening, discussions, and role playing, help the patient to cope adaptively (I)

Activity

Include the patient in decision-making activities (I)

Allow the patient realistic control over his or her hospitalization by allowing him or her to choose times for bathing, eating, ambulating, sitting in a chair, or visiting (I)

Allow the patient to talk with other people with the same diagnosis so that he or she can learn from others in a similar situation and can exchange information (I)

Place self-care items by the bedside so that the patient can provide care for him- or herself (I)

Pain

Administer prescribed analgesics (I)

Evaluate the presence of psychological pain associated with alterations in self-concept (I)

Bibliography

Carpenito, L. J. *Handbook of nursing diagnosis*. Philadelphia: Lippincott, 1984.

Gettrust, K., Ryan, S., & Engleman, D. *Applied nursing diagnosis*. New York: Wiley, 1985.

Gordon, M. *Manual of nursing diagnosis*. New York: McGraw-Hill, 1985.

Kim, M. J., McFarland, G., & McLane, A. *Nursing diagnosis*. St. Louis: C. V. Mosby, 1984.

Roberts, S. *Body image and self concept: Behavioral concepts and the criticall ill patient* (2nd ed.) Norwalk, Conn.: Appleton-Century-Crofts, 1986, pp. 379–405.

Rosenberg, M. & Kaplan, H. *Social psychology of the self concept*. Arlington Heights, Ill.: Harlan Davidson, Inc., 1982.

BODY-IMAGE DISTURBANCE

DEFINITION
Body image is the constantly changing total of conscious and unconscious information, feelings, and perceptions about one's body in space as different and apart from all others.

ETIOLOGY
Alteration in bodily integrity, including disfigurement
Unrealistic mental image of patient's own appearance
Inconsistence between perception of body image and reality
Failure to adapt to body-image alteration
Negation from others
Self-negation
Refusal to look at altered body part
Lack of participation in self-care
Social isolation
Threat of loss of body part
Dissociation of body from the disfiguring event
Physical immobility
Lack of knowledge

DEFINING CHARACTERISTICS

Regulatory Behaviors
Anorexia
Weight loss
Numbness of body part
Hypertension
Tachycardia
Tachypnea

Cognitive Behaviors
Fear of rejection
Anger
Hostility
Guilt
Shame
Withdrawal
Personalization of injured body part

Negative expression toward supportive devices
Depression
Restlessness
Altered spatial concept of self
Rejection of others
Denial of lost or altered body part
Alteration in body boundaries
Focus on altered or lost body part
Dependence
Refusal to accept change in self
Refusal to accept changes in lifestyle
Apathy
Hopelessness

NURSING RESPONSIBILITIES

Assessment

Assess the patient's prehospital perception of body image (I)
Assess situations contributing to perceptual change in body image (I)
Observe regulatory behaviors indicative of body-image disturbance (I)
Observe cognitive behaviors indicative of body-image disturbance (I)

Interventions

Fluid

Remove various supportive devices as soon as it is realistic to do so (I)

Aeration

Clarify for the patient his or her physical location in critical care and the location of his or her illness or injury (I)

Nutrition

Assist the patient with his or her diet (I)
Incorporate the patient's likes and dislikes into the diet, when possible (I)

Communication

Provide knowledge regarding biological change (I)

Listen to the patient's verbalization of alterations in body image (I)

Help the patient to match his or her perception of body image with reality (I)

Use simple explanations when describing the patient's illness, treatments, or progress (I)

Provide feedback as to how the altered body part is healing (I)

Assist the patient in developing coping mechanisms for body-image disturbance (I)

Help the patient to make realistic future goals (I)

Assist the patient in incorporating body changes into new or altered roles (I)

Activity

Encourage physical mobility or activity (I)

Encourage diversional activities (I)

Encourage the patient to participate in his or her own care (I)

Pain

Evaluate the type, location, and duration of pain (I)

Administer prescribed analgesics (D)

Bibliography

Gordon, M. *Manual of nursing diagnosis.* New York: McGraw-Hill, 1985.

Kim, M. J., McFarland, G., & McLane, A. *Nursing diagnosis.* St. Louis: C. V. Mosby, 1984.

Norris, C. The professional nurse and body image in Carlson, C. (ed.), *Behavioral concepts and nursing interventions.* Philadelphia: Lippincott, 1978, pp. 5–36.

Roberts, S. *Body image and self concept: Behavioral concepts and the critically ill patient* (2nd ed.). Norwalk, Conn.: Appleton-Century-Crofts, 1986, pp. 379–405.

FEAR OF SEPARATION

When the critically ill patient is admitted into critical care, he or she is most anxious about the threats to his or her biological well-being. The critical care unit[*] may represent biological security, but it does not represent emotional security.

ANXIETY

DEFINITION

An unpleasant emotional reaction that results from the perception of a particular situation as being threatening (Schwarzer, Vander Ploeg, & Spielberger, 1982).

OTHER DEFINITIONS

Transfer Anxiety

Anxiety experienced by the individual when he or she moves from a familiar, somewhat secure, environment to an environment that is unfamiliar and/or insecure.

Primary Anxiety

An elemental experience that, if it reaches a certain degree of intensity, is linked directly with the onset of defense mechanisms (Bowlby, 1960).

Expectant Anxiety

Defined as the point when an individual has reached a stage of development in which, to some degree of foresight, it becomes possible that he or she is able to predict situations as being dangerous and can take measures to avoid such situations (Bowlby, 1960).

ETIOLOGY

Threat of illness
Inconsistence between values and lifestyle changes
Unfamiliar environmental settings
Separation from family
Removal from familiar belongings
Fear of unknown
Inability to comprehend consequences of illness
Threat of death
Alteration in body image
Threat to self-concept
Obstruction of goals
Transfer within critical care

Insomnia
Speech pattern change

Cognitive Behaviors
Irritability
Aggressiveness
Confusion
Feeling of unreality
Restlessness

NURSING RESPONSIBILITIES

Assessment
Assess regulatory behaviors indicative of fear (I)
Assess cognitive behaviors indicative of fear (I)
Monitor ECG pattern continuously (I)
Assess prehospital situations in which the patient expressed
fear (I)
Observe hospital factors contributing to fear (I)
Auscultate the heart for rate, rhythm, and regularity (I)
Auscultate the chest for respiratory rate, rhythm, and regu-
larity (I)

Interventions

Fluid
Administer prescribed medications (D)
Measure intake, urinary volume, and specific gravity (I)
Measure arterial blood pressure (I)

Aeration
Administer humidified oxygen by mask, nasal catheter, or
nasal prongs at the prescribed flow rate (D)
Reduce meaningless environmental stimuli (I)
Evaluate the patient's breathing pattern for dyspnea (I)

Nutrition
Provide the patient with a prescribed diet (I)
Assist the patient with eating (I)
Consult with a dietitian (I)

Communication
Reduce the patient's fear regarding the critical care environment (I)

Listen to the patient's verbalization of his or her fears (I)

Help the patient to identify the source of his or her fears (I)

Instruct the patient regarding his or her role in critical care (I)

Provide knowledge regarding the patient's illness and treatment procedures (I)

Assist the patient in using available support systems (I)

Explore with the patient previous achievements or successes (I)

Activity

Encourage the patient to ambulate (I)

Provide diversional activities (I)

Pain

Administer prescribed analgesics (D)

Evaluate the type, location, and duration of pain (I)

Bibliography

Carpenito, L. J. *Handbook of nursing diagnosis.* Philadelphia: Lippincott, 1984.

Jones, P. & Jakob, D. Nursing Diagnosis: Differentiating fear from anxiety. *Nursing Papers*, 13, 20–29, Winter 1983.

Kim, M. J., McFarland, G., & McLane, A. *Nursing diagnosis.* St. Louis: C. V. Mosby, 1984.

Nikas, D., Stark, J., & Williams, S. *Core curriculum for critical care nursing.* Philadelphia: W. B. Saunders, 1981.

FEELING OF DEPRESSION

The critical care nurse can assess depression according to a general model of self-regulation involving three stages: self-monitoring, which consists of perception of loss and of life stressors; self-evaluation, which consists of a negative view of self, of experience, and of the future; and self-reinforcement.

DEPRESSION

DEFINITION

A manifestation of hopelessness felt in regard to the attainment of goals when responsibility for the hopelessness is attributed to one's personal deficit (Seligman, 1974).

ETIOLOGY
Medications
Endocrine disorders
Illness
Feelings of powerlessness
Perceived loss of body function, part or whole
Feelings of loneliness and inadequacy
Guilt
Loss perceived as punishment
Role changes
Lifestyle changes
Financial loss
Separation from significant others
Altered decision-making power
Negative view of self
Negative view of experiences
Failure to see progress in, or positive aspects of, illness
Negative view of future
Self-criticism
Threat to bodily integrity

DEFINING CHARACTERISTICS

Regulatory Behaviors
Anorexia
Weight loss
Indigestion
Dry mouth
Insomnia
Diurinal variations
Constipation
Diarrhea
Ulcers
Menstrual changes
Headaches
Tightness in chest
Tachycardia
Fatigue
Tiredness
Tension

Cognitive Behaviors
  Sadness
  Crying easily
  Sleep disturbance
  Social withdrawal
  Loss of feeling
  Boredom
  Indifference
  Lack of interest or motivation
  Self-criticism
  Avoidance
  Hopelessness
  Confusion
  Emptiness
  Irritability
  Memory loss
  Negativism
  Apathy
  Indecisiveness

NURSING RESPONSIBILITIES

Assessment

  Assess prehospital factors contributing to depression (I)
  Assess hospital events contributing to depression (I)
  Observe regulatory behaviors indicating depression (I)
  Observe cognitive behaviors indicating depression (I)
  Assess the effects of medication therapy (I)

Interventions

Fluid

  Provide knowledge regarding the patient's illness, treatment
    procedures, and progress (I)
  Provide knowledge regarding supportive devices attached to
    the patient (I)

Aeration

  Listen to the patient's verbalization of concerns regarding
    the illness, injury, or disease process (I)

Evaluate nonverbal cues for pain—facial grimace, tachy-cardia, tachypnea, and hypertension (I)

Consult with the physician regarding the patient's pain experience (I)

Activity

Provide distraction to decrease the intensity of pain and to increase the patient's tolerance to it (I)

Encourage physical mobility (I)

Encourage the patient to change his or her position (I)

Pain

Teach relaxation techniques to reduce pain (I)

Provide the patient with information regarding what to expect during a pain experience (I)

Bibliography

Carpenito, L. J. *Handbook of nursing diagnosis.* Philadelphia: Lippin-cott, 1984.

Gettrust, K., Ryan, S., & Engleman, D. *Applied nursing diagnosis.* New York: Wiley, 1985.

Gordon, M. *Manual of nursing diagnosis.* New York: McGraw-Hill, 1985

Kim, M. J., McFarland, G., & McLane, A. *Nursing diagnosis.* St. Louis: C. V. Mosby, 1984.

Kim, S. Pain: Theory, research and nursing practice. *Advances in Nursing Science*, 2, 43–59, January 1980.

Roberts, S. *Pain: Behavioral concepts and the critically ill patient* (2nd ed.). Norwalk, Conn.: Appleton-Century-Crofts, 1986, pp. 502–527.

Voshall, B. The effects of preoperative teaching on postoperative pain. *Topics in Clinical Nursing* 2, 39–43, April 1980.

Gettrust, K., Ryan, S., & Engleman, D. *Applied nursing diagnosis.* New York: Wiley, 1985.

Gordon, M. *Manual of nursing diagnosis.* New York: McGraw-Hill, 1985.

Kim, M. J., McFarland, G., & McLane, A. *Nursing diagnosis.* St. Louis: C. V. Mosby, 1984.

Mackinnon-Kesler, S. Maximizing your ICU patient's sensory and perceptual environment. *Canadian Nurse,* 79(5), 41–45, May 1983.

Roberts, S. *Sensory overload: Behavioral concepts and the critically ill patient.* (2nd ed.). Norwalk, Conn.: Appleton-Century-Crofts, 1986, pp. 332–355.

SENSORY DEPRIVATION

Sensory deprivation in critical care can also be called emotional–touch deprivation. Sensory deprivation is assessed according to its causes—reduction in stimulation of the senses, reduction in meaningfulness of stimulation, removal from familiar stimulation, and restrictions imposed on bodily movement.

DEFINITION
A combination of social isolation and reduced sensory stimulation leading to an environment providing little stimulus change (Wood, 1977).

OTHER DEFINITIONS
Technological Deprivation
In a highly technical environment dominated by machines, the patient loses precedence to the machine.

Perceptual Deprivation
The absence or reduction of stimulus variability is referred to as perceptual deprivation and occurs in an environment in which sound is muffled, light is diffused, and bodily sensations are nondistinct.

ETIOLOGY

Alterations in biological stability, including complications
Alterations in patient's ability to receive and interpret meaningful stimuli
- Neurological
- Chemical
- Cardiovascular
- Musculoskeletal

Understimulation of senses due to diagnostic or treatment modalities
- Tracheostomy tube
- Endotracheal tube
- Nasogastric tube
- Arterial line
- Peripheral lines
- Intracranial pressure monitoring
- Traction
- Casts
- Isolation
- Physical immobility
- Lack of patterning of environmental stimuli
- Meaningless stimuli from supportive devices
- Lack of knowledge
- Loss of control
- Underload of meaningful professional jargon
- Unfamiliarity in a highly technical environment
- Impaired communication

DEFINING CHARACTERISTICS

Regulatory Behaviors

Increased galvanic skin response
Minor itching
Increased catecholamines
Altered electroencephalogram patterns
Feeling excessively warm or cold
Muscle movement
Numbness in fingers and toes

Cognitive Behaviors

Visual and auditory hallucinations
Illusions

Temporal and spatial disorganization/disorientation
Inability to think clearly
Inability to concentrate
Anxiousness
Loss of sense of time
Delusions
Restlessness
Psychotic behavior
Noncompliant behavior
Confusion
Apathy
Depression
Dependence

NURSING RESPONSIBILITIES

Assessment

Assess prehospital factors contributing to feelings of deprivation (I)
Monitor environmental factors leading to sensory deprivation (I)
Assess critical care situations in which the patient experiences sensory deprivation (I)
Observe regulatory behaviors indicative of sensory deprivation (I)
Observe cognitive behaviors indicative of sensory deprivation (I)
Assess the patient's medications and their possible influence upon his or her sensory intake (I)

Interventions

Fluid

Provide knowledge regarding the meaning behind diagnostic and treatment modalities (I)
Provide meaningful touch (I)

Aeration

Provide clocks and calendars to foster orientation (I)
Provide an environment that keeps the patient human and functioning efficiently (I)
Surround the patient with familiar items from home and work (I)

Turn lights on during the day and off during sleeping hours (I)

Nutrition

Provide foods that stimulate the patient's senses (I)

Create a stimulating atmosphere conducive to eating (I)

Communication

Help the patient to incorporate changes occurring in the environment (I)

Assist the patient in controlling incoming stimuli (I)

Provide knowledge regarding data obtained from diagnostic or treatment modalities (I)

Discuss current events or events happening outside the patient's immediate environment (I)

Activity

Assist the family in providing meaningful interaction (I)

Reduce the degree and duration of territorial or spatial invasion (I)

Provide meaningful interaction between the critical care team and the patient (I)

Increase the use of meaningful stimuli—touch or contact between the patient's family and friends (I)

Encourage the patient to watch favorite television shows and news periodically throughout the day (I)

Organize nursing care to provide for adequate rest periods (I)

Provide the patient with his or her glasses, hearing aid, or dentures (I)

Pain

Administer analgesics to relieve pain (D)

Bibliography

Carpenito, L. J. *Handbook of nursing diagnosis.* Philadelphia: Lippincott, 1984.

Gordon, M. *Manual of nursing diagnosis.* New York: McGraw-Hill, 1985.

Kim, M. J., McFarland, G., & McLane, A. *Nursing diagnosis.* St. Louis: C. V. Mosby, 1984.

Kleck, H. ICU syndrome: Onset, manifestations, treatment, stressors, and prevention. *Critical Care Quarterly*, 6(4), 21–28, March 1984.

Roberts, S. *Sensory deprivation: Behavioral concepts and the critically ill patient* (2nd ed.). Norwalk, Conn.: Appleton-Century-Crofts, 1986, pp. 356–378.

Wood, M. Clinical sensory deprivation: A comparative study of patients in single care and two bed rooms. *Journal of Nursing Administration*, 7(10), 28–32, December 1977.

SLEEP PATTERN DISTURBANCE

The once-quiet patient may become an angry patient, throwing objects in his or her room or becoming confused. In critical care units, the nurse may have to awaken the patient every 1 to 2 hours in order to check the patient's vital signs, measure urine output, or perform a suctioning technique. Sleep deprivation, due to these (and other) factors, causes angry and confused behavior.

Sleep pattern disturbance is an overall category for specific sleep components, such as normal sleep, REM sleep, NREM sleep, and sleep deprivation.

DEFINITIONS

Sleep Pattern Disburbance
An alteration in the quality and/or quantity of sleep required by an individual so that he or she is unable to destructure the overcrowded data storage accumulated each day in critical care or to reinforce his or her character structure.

OTHER DEFINITIONS

Sleep
A mode of behavioral adaptation to the environment that is characterized as a behavioral state of diminished responsibility (Webb, 1983).

REM (Desynchronized Rapid Eye Movement) Sleep
Also called active or paradoxical sleep because of the high levels of neurological and general physiological activity. REM sleep is significant for learning, memory, and psychological adaptation (Wotring, 1982; Sebila, 1981; Hayter, 1980).

NREM (Synchronized Nonrapid Eye Movement) Sleep

Synchronized NREM is divided into four stages; its purpose is to restore the individual physically.

Sleep Deprivation

Lack of adequate sleep or dream time, related to prior or unusual sleep patterns (McFadden & Giblin, 1971, p. 249). Stage I represents a transition between the awake state and the sleep state. Stage II acts as a door between REM and NREM sleep and consists of a light sleep. Stage III is associated with deeper sleep and requires a louder noise to awaken the individual. Finally, stage IV signifies profound sleep, from which arousal is difficult (Roberts 1986).

ETIOLOGY

Excessive noise
Pain
Illness
Immobility
Anxiety
Stress
Medications
Lack of exercise
Depression
Fear of death
Loneliness
Being awakened for treatments and/or diagnostic procedures

DEFINING CHARACTERISTICS

Regulatory Behaviors

NREM sleep regulatory behaviors
    Decreased blood pressure
    Decreased heart rate
    Decreased respiratory rate
    Decreased urine volume
    Decreased plasma volume
    Decreased metabolic rate
    Decreased oxygen consumption
    Decreased carbon dioxide expiration
REM sleep regulatory behaviors
    Increased heart rate

Increased respiratory rate
Increased blood pressure
Increased autonomic activity
Increased metabolic activity
Increased gastric secretions
Increased 17-level hydrocortisone
Increased catecholamine level

Cognitive Behaviors
Lassitude
Lethargy
Hallucinations
Disorientation
Confusion
Restlessness
Irritability
Apathy
Poor judgment
Memory disturbance
Delusions
Paranoid ideation
Hostility

NURSING RESPONSIBILITIES

Assessment

Assess situations in which excess stimulation occurs (I)

Monitor time and length of time that a patient is awake at night (I)

Assess the patient's pre-illness sleep pattern and sleep history (I)

Assess the patient's pre-sleep night-time rituals (I)

Observe for behavior indicating that the patient is troubled and unable to sleep (I)

Inspect the patient's sleep pattern to determine whether or not he or she is in NREM or REM sleep (I)

Assess the effectiveness of night-time sedatives (I)

Assess cognitive behaviors indicative of alterations in sleep pattern (I)

Assess regulatory behaviors indicative of alterations in sleep pattern (I)

Interventions

Fluid

Provide sedatives as ordered (D)

Organize interventions around the patient's sleep cycle, when realistic (I)

Evaluate the patient's medications given in the evening to determine whether or not they could cause nightmares or hallucinations (I)

Limit fluid intake after 6:00 P.M. (I)

Instruct the patient to void as part of bedtime activity (I)

Aeration

Eliminate extraneous stimuli such as lights, unnecessary activities, noise, and staff verbal exchange, when realistic (I)

Position ventilator so that it produces the lowest decibel level for the patient (I)

Reduce machine alarm decibel to the lowest acceptable level (I)

Turn off suction and oxygen units when they are not in use (I)

Darken room at night and for naps (I)

Adjust room temperature and provide blankets for comfort (I)

Schedule treatments, including medications and respiratory therapy, prior to sleep (I)

Nutrition

Withhold beverages containing caffeine (I)

Avoid heavy meals before rest periods (I)

Provide a small snack before bedtime, if the patient desires (I)

Communication

Listen to the patient's concerns, fears, and anxieties (I)

Allow the patient to ventilate feelings before bedtime (I)

Activity

Provide daytime activity, such as range-of-motion exercises, sitting, standing, or walking (I)

Encourage the patient to increase his or her activity level during the day so that he or she can sleep at night (I)

Position the patient so that he or she is comfortable (I)

Provide meaningful touch through backrubs (I)

Evaluate and provide the patient's usual sleep stimuli, such as radio or television (I)

Allow the patient's spouse to sleep over in the patient's room (I)

Provide ear plugs to eliminate extraneous environmental stimuli, if necessary (I)

Pain

Evaluate whether or not pain is causing loss of sleep (I)

Bibliography

Carpenito, L. J. *Handbook of nursing diagnosis.* Philadelphia: Lippincott, 1984.

Chuman, M. A. The neurological basis of sleep. *Heart & Lung*, 12(2), 177–182, March 1983.

Croy, S. S. Sleep and sleep disorders: Normal sleep. *Professional Medical Assistant*, 16(1), 16–17, January–February 1983.

Gettrust, K., Ryan, S., & Engleman, D. *Applied nursing diagnosis.* New York: Wiley, 1985.

Helpenn-Synder, R. The effect of critical care unit noise on patient sleep cycle. *Critical Care Quarterly*, 7(4), 41–50, March 1985.

Hayter, J. The rhythm of sleep. *American Journal of Nursing*, 80, 457–461, March 1980.

Kim, M. J., McFarland, G., & McLane, A. *Nursing diagnosis.* St. Louis: C. V. Mosby, 1984.

Roberts, S. *Sleep deprivation: Behavioral concepts and the critically ill patient* (2nd ed.). Norwalk, Conn.: Appleton-Century-Crofts, 1986, pp. 63–94.

Sanford, S. Sleep and the cardiac patient. *Cardiovascular Nursing*, 19(5), 19–24, September–October 1983.

Sebilia, A. Sleep deprivation and biological rhythms in the critical care unit. *Critical Care Nursing*, 19–23, May–June 1981.

Webb, W. Theories in modern sleep research in Mayes, A. (ed.), *Sleep Mechanism and functions*, Cambridge, Mass.: Van Nostrand Reinhold, 1983, pp. 1–17.

Wotring, K. Using research in practice. *Focus*, 34–36, October–November 1982

STRESS

Stress affects all critically ill patients. Hospitalization due to a biophysiological illness can create both physiological and psychological stress.

DEFINITION

An intense exertion being experienced by the individual in response to stimuli that eventually tax the physiological, psychological, or sociological systems.

OTHER DEFINITIONS

Stressors

Agents or factors that challenge the adaptive capacities of an individual, thereby placing a strain upon that person which may result in stress and/or disease.

Stages of Stress

There are three stages of stress. They are: (1) *the alarm stage*, which implies, with disease, illness, or injury, that there is a fight to maintain the homeostatic balance of the individual tissues when they are damaged; (2) *the stage of resistance or adaptation*, which is characterized by the lessening of the initial symptoms associated with the alarm reaction, so that the individual can prepare for the next crisis; and (3) *the stage of exhaustion*, which implies that the body is exposed to noxious stimuli for a prolonged period of time, causing the body to lose its acquired ability to resist, thus becoming exhausted.

ETIOLOGY

> Threat phase of illness, in which death is a possibility
> Unfamiliar and technical environment
> Threat of invasive procedures
> Loss of biological integrity
> Separation from significant others
> Dependence upon strangers
> Loss of control to supportive devices
> Lack of decision-making power

Threat of complications
Excess sensory stimuli
Anger
Depression
Loss of employment
Altered lifestyle
Financial loss
Lack of knowledge
Insecurity with the future
Obstructed goals
Perception of illness incongruent with reality
Limited external resources

DEFINING CHARACTERISTICS

Regulatory Behaviors
Increased heart rate
Increased myocardial contraction
Increased coronary vasoconstriction
Increased general vasoconstriction
Increased blood pressure
Pupil dilation
Increased serum glucose
Bronchiolar dilation
Increased cardiac output
Decreased urinary output
Dyspnea
Shortness of breath
Gastric discomfort
Hand tremors
Muscle tension
Diaphoresis
Palpitation

Cognitive Behaviors
Anxiety
Fear
Increased mental activity
Abnormal head movement
Irrelevant or constant conversation

    Restlessness
    Agitation
    Fatigue
    Increase in errors
    Reduced objective thinking
    Reduced adaptive efficiency
    Sarcasm
    Negativism
    Inappropriate humor

NURSING RESPONSIBILITIES

Assessment

Assess degree and duration of stress as it pertains to the patient's illness, injury, or disease process (I)

Assess the patient's prehospital stress-coping strategies (I)

Monitor statements and situations that contribute to stress (I)

Observe regulatory behaviors indicating stress reaction (I)

Observe cognitive behaviors indicating stress reactions (I)

Interventions

Fluid

Instruct the patient as to the meaning of his or her biological illness (I)

Explain the purpose behind supportive devices or treatment procedures (I)

Aeration

Minimize environmental stressors, such as noise or lights (I)

Provide privacy (I)

Nutrition

Create a stress-free environment that is conducive to eating (I)

Communication

Help the patient to identify alternate ways of coping with stress (I)

Help the patient to identify environmental or situational factors contributing to stress (I)

Listen to the patient's verbalization of fears and anxieties related to his or her illness or disease (I)

Encourage family support and participation in care (I)

Identify the patient's perception of his or her illness and role as a patient (I)

Clarify any misconceptions regarding illness, treatments, and/or progress (I)

Discuss with the patient his or her previous hospital and illness experiences (I)

Assist the patient in making realistic future goals (I)

Facilitate communication between the patient and his or her friends (I)

Activity

Teach relaxation techniques (I)

Encourage interdependence and eventual independence (I)

Encourage the patient to participate in his or her care and decision making (I)

Help the patient to identify external resources (I)

Pain

Evaluate whether or not the patient's pain is due to stress (I)

Bibliography

DeViller, B. Physiology of stress: Cellular healing. *Critical Care Quarterly*, 6(4), 15-20, March 1984.

Guzzetta, C. & Forsyth, G. Nursing diagnostic pilot study: Psychophysiological stress. *Advance in Nursing Science*, 1, 27-44, 1979.

Lippincott, R. Psychological stress factors in decision making. *Heart & Lung*, 8(6), 1093-1097, November-December 1979

Luckman, J. & Sorensen, K. Stress and disease: Major causative factors. *Medical-surgical nursing: A psychophysiological approach*. Philadelphia: W. B. Saunders, 1974, pp. 41-47.

Pollock, S. The stress response. *Critical Care Quarterly*, 6(4), 1-14, March 1984.

Roberts, S. *Stress: Behavioral concepts and the critically ill patient* (2nd ed.). Norwalk, Conn.: Appleton-Century-Crofts, 1986, pp. 406-430.

Selye, H. A code for coping with stress. *AORN Journal*, 25(1), 35-42, January 1977.

Williams, S. Physiological aspects of stress. *Australian Nurses Journal*, 9, 44-48, July 1979.

6

Physiological Assessment

Having assessed the critically ill patient's behavioral, emotional, and environmental system, and having formulated nursing diagnosis, the nurse begins the sometimes tedious task of making physiological assessments.

CARDIOVASCULAR SYSTEM

The critical care nurse uses his or her expertise in physical assessment to gather data, formulate a collaborative cardiac-related nursing diagnosis, and delineated appropriate interventions.

CARDIAC PRESSURES, ALTERATION IN

Alteration in Right Ventricular–Atrial Preload

DEFINITION
Right ventricular preload is measured by central venous pressure (CVP) or right atrial pressure and reflects changes in right ventricular pressure. It involves measuring both blood volume and quality of central venous return.

ETIOLOGY
　　Low right ventricular reload (CVP)
　　　　Hemorrhage

Sepsis
Vasodilatation (anaphylactic shock)
High right ventricular preload (CVP)
Cor pulmonale
Pulmonary hypertension
Right atrial myxoma
Tamponade
Chronic obstructive pulmonary disease
Hypoxia leading to pulmonary vasoconstriction
Pulmonary infections
Tricuspid insufficiency
Tricuspid stenosis
Right intracardiac shunt
Overinfusion of IV fluid
Right ventricular myocardial infarction
Constrictive pericarditis

DEFINING CHARACTERISTICS

Regulatory Behaviors
Hepatomegaly
Ascites
Positive hepatojugular reflux
Cool extremities
Cyanosis of nail beds
Distended jugular veins
Peripheral or dependent edema
Increased CVP
S_3 (ventricular gallop)
S_4 (atrial gallop)
Pansystolic or holosystolic murmur
Abdominal fullness
Vomiting
Anorexia
Nausea

Cognitive Behaviors
Fatigue
Weakness
Lack of interest in activities

NURSING RESPONSIBILITIES

Assessment

Assess regulatory behaviors indicative of alteration in right ventricular preload (I)

Assess cognitive behaviors indicative of alteration in right ventricular preload (I)

Monitor right ventricular pressure (I)

Assess the effectiveness of prescribed medications (I)

Monitor cardioscope and ECG for arrhythmias (I)

Auscultate the heart for abnormal heart sounds (I)

Auscultate the heart for rate, rhythm, and regularity (I)

Auscultate the chest for adventitious breath sounds (I)

Auscultate the chest for respiratory rate, rhythm, and regularity (I)

Interventions

Fluid

Administer prescribed medications used to decrease preload (D)

Dopamine
Digitalis
Pronestyl
Propranolol
Quinidine
Lasix

Administer the prescribed IV fluids (D)

Measure blood pressure and mean arterial pressure (MAP)

Measure blood pressure and MAP (I)

Evaluate data from hemodynamic parameters: pulmonary artery pressure (PAP), pulmonary capillary wedge pressure (PCWP), systemic vascular resistance (SVR), CVP, and cardiac output (CO)

Evaluate the jugular veins for distension (I)

Evaluate the skin for color, temperature, and presence of diaphoresis (I)

Aeration

Administer humidified oxygen at the prescribed flow rate (D)

Reduce meaningless environmental stimuli (I)
Evaluate arterial blood gasses (I)

Nutrition
Provide the prescribed low-salt diet (D)
Assist the patient with eating (I)

Communication
Listen to the patient's concerns, fears, and frustrations (I)
Reduce the patient's anxiety level (I)
Provide knowledge regarding the causes of elevated right
   ventricular preload (I)
Inform the physician of any changes in the patient's status
   (I)

Activity
Alternate rest and moderate activity periods (I)
Encourage the use of diversional activities (I)
Teach the patient passive range-of-motion exercises (I)

Pain
Administer prescribed analgesics (D)
Evaluate the type, location, and duration of pain (I)

Bibliography

Johanson, B., Dungca, C., Hoffmeister, D., & Wells, S. *Standards for
   critical care.* (2nd ed.). St. Louis: C. V. Mosby, 1985.
Roberts, S. *Physiological concepts and the critically ill.* Englewood
   Cliffs, N.J.: Prentice-Hall, 1985, pp. 1–54; 55–100.

Alterations in Left Ventricular–Atrial Preload

DEFINITION
The length to which myocardial fibers are stretched at the end
of diastole, whereby an increase in the preload causes an increase in the tension of myocardial muscle, increased force of
contraction, and increased stroke volume.

ETIOLOGY
    Low left ventricular–atrial preload
        Hemorrhage
        Vasodilatation
            Medication
                Nitroprusside
        Anaphylactic shock
        Neurogenic shock
    High left ventricular–atrial preload
        Overinfusion of IV fluids
        Atrial or ventricular septal deficit
        Left ventricular myocardial infarction
        Left ventricular aneurysm
        Hypoxemia
        Metabolic acidosis
        Hypoperfusion of the heart
        Increased peripheral vascular resistance due to:
            Cold
            Drugs
                Epinephrine
                Norepinephrine
                Aramine
        Left atrial myxoma
        Aortic insufficiency
        Aortic stenosis
        Coarctation of aorta
        Pulmonary embolism
        Positive and expiratory pressure (PEEP) or continuous
            positive airway pressure (CPAP)
        Ventilator
        Pneumothorax

DEFINING CHARACTERISTICS

Regulatory Behaviors
    Tachycardia
    Pulsus alternans
    Dusky to ashen skin color

S_3 (ventricular gallop)
Syncope
Dyspnea
Cheyne–Stokes
Rales or wheezes
Decreased urinary output
Nocturia
Pink-tinged mucus

Cognitive Behaviors
Disorientation
Incoherent speech
Restlessness
Weakness
Confusion
Impaired decision-making ability

NURSING RESPONSIBILITIES

Assessment
Assess regulatory behaviors indicative of alteration in left
ventricular preload (I)
Assess cognitive behaviors indicative of alteration in left
ventricular preload (I)
Monitor the ECG pattern continuously (I)
Observe the side or therapeutic effects of prescribed medi-
cations (I)
Auscultate the heart for abnormal heart sounds, such as S_4
and S_3 (I)
Palpate the apical impulse, noting its position and quality
(I)
Auscultate the chest for adventitious breath sounds (I)
Auscultate the chest for respiratory rate, rhythm, and
regularity (I)

Interventions

Fluids
Administer prescribed medications (D)
Dopamine
Nitroprusside

Dobutamine
Pronestyl
Lasix
Evaluate PAP and PCWP pressures (I)
PAP
Normal 25/10 mmHg
Pulmonary artery diastolic pressure (10 mmHg) approximates the left ventricular end diastolic pressure (LVEDP) or pulmonary capillary wedge pressure (PCWP)
PCWP
Normal: 10–12 mmHg
PCWP indirectly reflects left atrial pressure
Evaluate CVP, CO, and SVR (I)
Administer IV fluids as ordered to prevent overinfusion and elevated preload (D)
Measure CVP, PAP, PCWP, and CO q1h or as needed (I)
Measure blood pressure and pulse q1h or as needed for hypotension, pulsus alternans, and tachycardia (I)
Measure intake, urinary volume, and specific gravity (I)

Aeration

Administer oxygen as ordered, via mask, nasal catheter, or nasal prongs (D)
Reduce meaningless environmental stimuli (I)

Nutrition

Provide the prescribed diet (D)
Consult with the dietitian (I)
Assist the patient with his or her diet (I)

Communication

Provide knowledge regarding drugs used to decrease pre-load (I)
Provide knowledge regarding the use of Swan-Ganz to monitor PAP and PCWP (I)
Reduce the patient's anxiety regarding the use of invasive diagnostic procedures (I)
Reduce the patient's anxiety related to causes of altered left ventricular–atrial preload (I)

Inform the physician of any changes in PAP or PCWP reflecting alteration in left ventricular–atrial preload (I)

Activity

Support the position (flat–45-degree angle) that will achieve best PAP and PCWP readings (I)

Support the position that provides the best comfort for the patient yet has the least effect upon an altered left ventricular–atrial preload (I)

Restrict physical activity that increases left ventricular–atrial preload (I)

Pain

Evaluate the type, location, and duration of any pain experienced by the patient (I)

Administer prescribed analgesics (D)

Bibliography

Johanson, B., Dungca, C., Hoffmeister, D., & Wells, S. *Standards for critical care* (2nd ed.). St. Louis: C. V. Mosby, 1985.

Laulive, J. Pulmonary artery pressure and position changes in the critically ill adult. *Dimension of Critical Care Nursing*, 1(1), 28–34, January–February 1982.

Roberts, S. *Physiological concepts and the critically ill patient.* Englewood Cliffs, N.J.: Prentice-Hall, 1985, pp. 1–54; 55–100.

Sedlock, S. Interpretation of hemodynamic pressures and recognition of complications. *Critical Care Nurse*, 39–54, November–December 1980.

Woods, S. & Mansfield, L. Effect of body position upon pulmonary artery and pulmonary capillary wedge pressures in noncritically ill patients. *Heart & Lung*, 5(1), 83–90, January–February 1976.

Alteration in Systemic Vascular Resistance, Afterload

DEFINITION

Afterload is defined as the amount of resistance against which the ventricle ejects its contents. As afterload increases, there is less volume ejected, leading to decreased stroke volume.

ETIOLOGY

Atherosclerosis

Hypertension

Aortic stenosis
Coarctation of the aorta
Vasoconstriction
Medications
    Epinephrine
    Norepinephrine
    Aramine
    Dopamine (high dose)
Ventricular dilatation
    Extreme cold
    Cardiogenic shock
    Left ventricular failure

DEFINING CHARACTERISTICS

Regulatory Behaviors
Cool extremities
Skin-color changes
Oliguria
Pallor and cyanosis
Tachypnea
Tachycardia
Dyspnea
Increased PCWP
Increased CVP
Weakness
Fatigue

Cognitive Behaviors
Pain
Decreased interest in environment
Irritability
Anxiety
Apathy
Lethargy
Confusion

NURSING RESPONSIBILITIES

Assessment
Assess regulatory behaviors indicative of alteration in systemic vascular resistance or afterload (I)

Assess cognitive behaviors indicative of alteration in systemic vascular resistance or afterload (I)

Monitor the ECG pattern continuously (I)

Assess the effects of prescribed medications (I)

Palpate the apical impulse, noting position and quality (I)

Auscultate the heart for abnormal heart sounds (I)

Auscultate the heart for rate, rhythm, and regularity (I)

Auscultate the chest for adventitious breath sounds (I)

Auscultate the chest for respiratory rate, rhythm, and regularity (I)

Intervention

Fluid

Administer IV fluids as prescribed (D)

Administer medications used to decrease afterload (D)

Nitroprusside

Dopamine

Dobutamine

Obtain necessary laboratory studies that will facilitate diagnosis (ID)

Evaluate for signs and symptoms of decreased perfusion, such as diaphoresis, cool skin, restlessness, confusion, and Chenye-Stokes respiration (I)

Regulate the IV flow rate and check for patency (I)

Measure systemic vascular resistance (I)

$$SVR = \frac{MAP - CVP}{CO}$$

$$MAP = Systolic - Diastolic - 3 + Diastolic$$

Measure intake, urinary volume, and specific gravity (I)

Aeration

Administer humidified oxygen at the prescribed flow rate (D)

Reduce unnecessary environmental stimuli (I)

Nutrition

Assist the patient with eating (I)

Incorporate the patient's food preferences into his or her diet, when possible (I)

Communication

    Reduce the patient's anxiety regarding invasive supportive procedures, such as intra-aortic balloon pump (IABP), arterial line, or Swan-Ganz (I)

    Provide knowledge regarding the purpose behind counter-pulsation (I)

    Reduce anxiety regarding the cause of altered systemic vascular resistance or afterload (I)

    Inform the physician of any changes in hemodynamic stability (I)

Activity

    Reduce afterload reduction through counterpulsation by IABP or cardioassist (D)

    Measure blood pressure, pulse, urinary output, CVP, PAP, and PCWP while the patient is on IABP (I)

    Auscultate cardiac sounds for any deviations (I)

    Measure any blood loss from the insertion site and report the loss to the physician (I)

    Support the patient through the use of hemodynamic supportive devices (I)

    Provide diversional activity while the patient is on counter-pulsation (I)

    Evaluate the patient while on IABP or counterassist, which includes timing for balloon inflation, checking calibration and timing of balloon inflation and deflation q1h, and checking for the presence of augmented pressure wave for placement and timing (I)

    Evaluate the safety of the patient while on counter pulsation (I)

Pain

    Evaluate the type, location, and duration of pain (I)

    Administer prescribed analgesics (I)

Bibliography

Johanson, B., Dungca, C., Hoffmeister, D., & Wells, S. *Standards for critical care* (2nd ed.). St. Louis: C. V. Mosby, 1985.

Roberts, S. *Physiological concepts and the critically ill patient.* Englewood Cliffs, N.J.: Prentice-Hall, 1985, pp. 1–54; 55–100.

Scholz, H. Inotropic drugs in the treatment of heart failure. *Hospital Practice*, 57–71, May 1984.

Alteration in Pulmonary Vascular Resistance, Afterload

DEFINITION
Pulmonary vascular resistance (PVR) is sometimes referred to as pulmonary arteriolar resistance. It is a measure of the pulmonary blood vessel resistance to blood flow, as well as an indicator of right ventricular afterload (Bustin, 1986).

ETIOLOGY
    High PVR
        Pulmonary hypertension
        Hypoxia
        Lung disease
        Pulmonary embolism
    Low pulmonary vascular resistance
        Septic shock
        Neurogenic shock
        Medications
            Nitroprusside
            Nitroglycerin
            Calcium antagonist

DEFINING CHARACTERISTICS

Regulatory Behaviors
    Shortness of breath
    Tachypnea
    Dyspnea
    Cyanosis
    Tachycardia
    Peripheral edema
    Increased CVP

Cognitive Behaviors
    Anxiousness
    Restlessness
    Confusion

NURSING RESPONSIBILITIES

Assessment
    Assess factors contributing to altered PVR (I)

Assess regulatory behaviors indicative of altered PVR (I)
Assess cognitive behaviors indicative of altered PVR resistance (I)
Monitor the ECG continuously (I)
Auscultate the heart for abnormal heart sounds (I)
Auscultate the heart for rate, rhythm, and regularity (I)
Auscultate the chest for adventitious breath sounds (I)
Auscultate the chest for respiratory rate, rhythm, and regularity (I)

Interventions

Fluid

Administer prescribed medications depending upon whether pulmonary vascular resistance is increased or decreased (D)
    Dilators
        Nitroprusside
        NTG
    Vasopressors
        Epinephrine
        Norepinephrine
        Dopamine
Measure pulmonary vascular resistance (I)

$$\frac{\text{Mean pulmonary arterial pressure (PAM)} - \text{PCWP}}{\text{CO}} \times 80$$

Obtain data for hemodynamic parameters: PCWP, PAP, CVP, CO, SVR, and PVR (I)
Evaluate for signs and symptoms of increased or decreased PVR (I)
Measure intake, output, and specific gravity (I)

Aeration

Administer humidified oxygen at the prescribed flow rate (I)
Evaluate the patient's tolerance of ventilatory support (I)
Suction the patient as needed (I)
Reduce unnecessary environmental stimuli (I)

Nutrition

Assist the patient with eating (I)
Encourage the patient to maintain the prescribed diet (I)

Communication

Reduce the patient's anxiety regarding the invasive supportive procedure of an intra-aortic balloon pump (IABP) (I)

Provide knowledge regarding the purpose behind counterpulsation (I)

Inform the physician of any changes in the patient's PVR (I)

Activity

Reduce afterload through counterpulsation by means of an
IABP or cardioassist (D)

Measure blood pressure, pulse, urinary output, CVP, PAP,
PCWP, SVR, and PVR while the patient is on the IABP (I)

Provide diversional activity while the patient is on counterpulsation (I)

Pain

Evaluate the type, location, and duration of pain (I)

Administer prescribed analgesics (I)

Bibliography

Bustin, D. *Hemodynamic monitoring for critical care.* Norwalk, Conn.:
Appleton-Century-Crofts, 1986.

Urban, N. Integrating hemodynamic parameters with clinical decision-
making. *Critical Care Nurse*, 6(2), 48–61

CARDIAC OUTPUT, ALTERATION IN

Cardiac Output, Decreased

DEFINITION

Cardiac output is the volume of blood ejected by the left
ventricle in 1 minute; decreased cardiac output is inadequate
to meet the metabolic needs of the body's tissues.

ETIOLOGY

Acute myocardial infarction

Valvular disease

Aortic

Mitral

Tricuspid

Pulmonary

Cardiomyopathy

Hypertension
Arrhythmias
Cor pulmonale
Right ventricular infarction
Myocarditis
Ruptured chordae
Congestive heart failure
Cardiogenic shock
Chronic obstructive pulmonary disease
Diabetes mellitus
Adrenocortical insufficiency
Polycythemia
Anemia
Shock
Sepsis
Surgery
Medication
    Vasodilators
    Vasoconstrictors
Hypothermia
Hyperthermia

DEFINING CHARACTERISTICS

Regulatory Behaviors
Hypotension
Bradyarrhythmias
Tachyarrhythmias
Angina
Fatigue
Weakness
Jugular vein distension
Increased PAP
Increased PCWP
Increased SVR
Oliguria
Color changes of skin mucous membrane
Decreased peripheral pulse
Cold and clammy skin
Adventitious breath sounds, rales
Dyspnea

Orthopnea
Vertigo
Syncope
Decreased activity tolerance
Weight gain
Gallop rhythm

Cognitive Behaviors
Confusion
Restlessness
Anxiety
Stress
Fear

NURSING RESPONSIBILITIES

Assessment
Assess regulatory behaviors indicative of decreased cardiac output (I)
Assess cognitive behaviors indicative of decreased cardiac output (I)
Monitor the ECG for arrhythmias (I)
Monitor the side effects of medications prescribed for decreased cardiac output (I)
Assess the effectiveness of prescribed medications (I)
Assess the patient's neurological status q shift and prn (I)
Auscultate the heart for abnormal heart sounds: S_4 and S_3, splitting of heart sounds, abnormally loud or diminished beats, and point of maximal intensity (PMI) (I)
Auscultate the chest for adventitious breath sounds (I)

Interventions

Fluid
Administer medications used to increase cardiac output (D)
Dopamine
Dobutamine
Isuprel
Initiate IV therapy as ordered by the physician (ID)
Assist the physician in inserting central lines (ID)
Provide standardized care and observation of pulmonary artery catheter and insertion site, noting redness or

swelling at insertion site, appropriateness of waveform, and patency (ID)

Provide aseptic dressing change of pulmonary artery line and CVP line as ordered (ID)

Obtain vital signs q1–2h or as necessary (I)

Measure CVP, PAP, PCWP, and CO, and report any significant changes to the physician (I)

Measure intake, weight, and urinary output (I)

Regulate IV therapy according to unit protocol or physician order (I)

Maintain skin integrity for the patient who is on complete bed rest (I)

Regulate the flow rate of IV medications (I)

Measure cardiac output and cardiac index, if applicable (I)

Evaluate pulses, noting deviations such as pulse deficits, pulses alternans, water-hammer pulse, and pulse paradoxus (I)

Evaluate blood urea nitrogen (BUN), serum electrolytes, creatinine, complete blood cell count (CBC), and cardiac enzymes q shift and prn (I)

Aeration

Provide oxygen via mask, nasal catheter, or nasal prongs at the prescribed flow rate (D)

Obtain arterial blood gasses (ID)

Interpret blood gasses and report results to the physician (I)

Encourage the patient to cough, turn, and deep-breathe (I)

Provide an atmosphere conducive to adequate sleep and rest (I)

Minimize excessive meaningful stimuli (I)

Nutrition

Provide nutritional replacement appropriate for the patient's needs (I)

Communication

Reduce the patient's anxiety regarding the cause of decreased CO and behavioral responses (I)

Provide knowledge regarding diagnosis and supportive devices (I)

Encourage the patient to express concerns, fears, and anxieties (I)

Activity

Assist the physician in the insertion and care of the patient on an IABP (ID)

Limit strenuous physical activity (I)

Encourage patient participation in self-care (I)

Maintain proper positioning (I)

Pain

Evaluate the type, location, and duration of pain (I)

Evaluate for the presence of pain (I)

Bibliography

Carpenito, L. J. *Handbook of nursing diagnosis.* Philadelphia: Lippincott, 1984.

Gettrust, K., Ryan, S., & Engleman, D. *Applied nursing diagnosis.* New York: Wiley, 1985.

Gordon, M. *Manual of nursing diagnosis.* New York: McGraw-Hill, 1985.

Kim, M. J., McFarland, G., & McLane, A. *Nursing diagnosis.* St. Louis: C. V. Mosby, 1984.

Roberts, S. *Physiological concepts and the critically ill patient.* Englewood Cliffs, N.J. Prentice-Hall, 1985, pp. 55–100.

Wessel, S. & Kim, M. J. Nursing functions related to the nursing diagnosis, decreased cardiac output, in Kim, M. J., McFarland, G., & McLane, A. (eds.), *Classification of nursing diagnosis.* St. Louis: C. V. Mosby, 1984, pp. 192–198.

Cardiac Output, Increased

DEFINITION

Increased cardiac output is defined as a clinical situation in which circulation remains vigorous and the extremities remain warm.

ETIOLOGY

Congestive heart failure

Hyperthyroidism

Paget's disease

Anemia

Beriberi

Arteriovenous fistula

Increased physical activity

Fever
Tachycardia
Pulmonary edema

DEFINING CHARACTERISTICS

Regulatory Behaviors
Weight loss
Diaphoresis
Heat intolerance
Diarrhea
Arrhythmias
Tremor
Increased appetite
Calf tenderness
Increased venous pressure
Dyspnea

Cognitive Behaviors
Restlessness
Nervousness
Irritability
Fatigue

NURSING RESPONSIBILITIES

Assessment
Assess regulatory behaviors indicative of increased cardiac
output (I)
Assess cognitive behaviors indicative of increased cardiac
output (I)
Monitor the ECG for arrhythmias (I)
Assess the effects of medications, including side effects (I)
Auscultate the chest for adventitious breath sounds (I)

Interventions

Fluid
Administer prescribed medications (D)
Initiate IV therapy (D)
Regulate the IV flow rate and check for patency (I)
Measure vital signs (I)

Measure CVP, PAP, PCWP, and CO (I)

Measure intake, urinary volume, and specific gravity (I)

Aeration

Administer oxygen at the prescribed flow rate (D)

Provide an environment conducive to sleep and rest (I)

Nutrition

Encourage the patient to eat the prescribed diet (I)

Assist the patient with his or her diet (I)

Communication

Reduce anxiety regarding the causes of increased cardiac output (I)

Provide knowledge regarding invasive supportive or diagnostic procedures (I)

Reports to the physician changes in regulatory or cognitive behaviors indicative of increased cardiac output (I)

Activity

Limit physical activity (I)

Pain

Administer prescribed analgesics (D)

Evaluate the type, location, and duration of pain (I)

Bibliography

Roberts, S. *Physiological concepts and the critically ill patient.* Englewood Cliffs, N.J.: Prentice-Hall, 1985, pp. 55–100.

ARTERIAL BLOOD PRESSURE, ALTERATION IN

Arterial Blood Pressure Altered, Hypotension

DEFINITION

Hypotension is an abnormal fall in both systolic and diastolic arterial blood pressure.

ETIOLOGY

Hypoadrenergic orthostatic hypotension

Bradbury-Eggleton syndrome

Shy-Drager syndrome

       Diabetes mellitus
       End-stage renal disease
       Polyneuropathy
       Guillain-Barré syndrome
       Intracranial tumor
       Spinal cord tumor
       Cerebral infarction
       Neoplasm
       Alcoholism
       Surgical sympathectomy
    Hyperadrenergic orthostatic hypotension
       Hypovolemia
       Decreased venous tone or function
       Defective volume regulation
       Medications
          Antihypertensives
          Nitrates
          Calcium channel blockers
          Antidepressants
          Diuretics

DEFINING CHARACTERISTICS

Regulatory Behaviors
    Cool and clammy skin
    Oliguria
    Pallor
    Tachycardia
    Weak, thready pulse

Cognitive Behaviors
    Restlessness
    Confusion
    Agitation
    Lethargy
    Obtundation

NURSING RESPONSIBILITIES

Assessment
    Assess regulatory behaviors indicative of hypotension (I)
    Assess cognitive behaviors indicative of hypotension (I)

Monitor the ECG for arrhythmias (I)

Assess the side or therapeutic effects of prescribed medications (I)

Auscultate the heart for abnormal heart sounds, S_3 and S_4 (I)

Auscultate the chest for adventitious breath sounds (I)

Interventions

Fluid

Administer prescribed medications (D)

Initiate IV therapy (D)

Measure vital signs (I)

Measure CVP, PAP, PCWP, and CO (I)

Measure intake and urinary output volume (I)

Regulate the IV flow rate (I)

Aeration

Provide oxygen via mask, nasal cannula, or nasal prongs at the prescribed flow rate (D)

Create an environment conducive to sleep and rest (I)

Nutrition

Provide nutrition adequate to meet the patient's metabolic needs (ID)

Provide spiritual consultation as requested by the patient (I)

Communication

Listen to the patient's expression of fears, anxieties, or concerns (I)

Provide knowledge regarding the causes of hypotension (I)

Provide knowledge regarding the use of invasive diagnostic procedures and supportive devices (I)

Include the family in the patient's care (I)

Activity

Prevent postural changes that will reduce arterial blood pressure (I)

Minimize physical activity that will alter blood pressure stability (I)

Encourage diversional activities while the patient is on bed rest (I)

Pain
   Administer prescribed analgesics (D)
   Minimize discomfort from the underlying cause of hypotension (I)

Bibliography

Horowitz, L. & Groves, B. *Signs and symptoms in cardiology.* Philadelphia: Lippincott, 1985.

Arterial Blood Pressure Altered, Hypertension

DEFINITION
Hypertension is an elevated arterial blood pressure (160/95 mmHg).

ETIOLOGY
   Intravascular hypernatremia
   Obesity
   Increased dietary hypernatremia
   Atherosclerosis
   Renovascular hypertension
   Chronic renal insufficiency
   Chronic renal failure
   Renal transplantation
   Acute renal failure
   Renal hemangiopericytoma
   Juxtaglomerular cell tumor
   Wilms' tumor
   Clear cell carcinoma of the kidney
   Mineralocorticoid excess
   Primary aldosteronism
   Pheochromocytoma
   Oral contraceptive
   Coarctation of the aorta
   Cushing's syndrome
   Primary hyperthyroidism

DEFINING CHARACTERISTICS

Regulatory Behaviors
   Headache

Pallor
Nausea
Vomiting
Blurred vision
Fleeting numbness or tingling in the limb
Convulsion

Cognitive Behaviors
Nervousness
Irritability
Drowsiness
Confusion

NURSING RESPONSIBILITIES

Assessment
Assess regulatory behaviors indicative of hypertension (I)
Assess cognitive behaviors indicative of hypertension (I)
Monitor the side and therapeutic effects of prescribed medications (I)
Monitor the ECG for arrhythmias (I)
Auscultate the heart for abnormal heart sounds, S_4, and S_3 (I)

Interventions

Fluid
Administer prescribed antihypertensive medications and diuretics (D)
Obtain laboratory studies (D)
Start IV therapy once it has been ordered (I)
Regulate the IV flow rate, including medications (I)
Measure arterial blood pressure, pulse, and MAP (I)
Measure CVP, PAP, PCWP, and CO (I)
Measure intake and urinary volume (I)
Interpret laboratory results and inform the physician of significant changes (I)

Aeration
Provide oxygen via mask, nasal catheter, or nasal cannula at the prescribed flow rate (D)
Encourage coughing, turning, and deep breathing (I)
Encourage the patient to stop smoking (I)

Nutrition

Encourage the patient to eat the prescribed low-sodium diet (I)

Assist the patient with eating (I)

Provide a spiritual support system (I)

Encourage the patient's participation in a weight-reduction program (I)

Communication

Encourage communication between patient–family–staff (I)

Reduce meaningless environmental stimuli (I)

Listen to the patient's concerns regarding role changes (I)

Reduce the patient's anxiety regarding the causes of hypertension (I)

Encourage participation in relaxation exercises (I)

Listen to the patient's concerns regarding possible financial reversal due to illness (I)

Activity

Encourage physical mobility through exercise (I)

Provide diversional activity (I)

Pain

Administer prescribed medications (D)

Encourage the patient to describe the pain experience: location, type, onset, duration, and precipitating events (I)

Bibliography

Horowitz, L. & Groves, B. *Signs and symptoms in cardiology.* Philadelphia: Lippincott, 1985.

TISSUE PERFUSION, ALTERATION IN
Coronary Artery Perfusion, Decreased

DEFINITION

Decreased coronary artery perfusion implies reduced blood flow through the right and/or left coronary arteries, which provide the entire blood supply to the myocardium.

ETIOLOGY

Arteriosclerosis

Aortic stenosis

    Coronary artery spasm
    Ischemic heart disease
    Hypovolemia
    Trauma
    Acute myocardial infarction

DEFINING CHARACTERISTICS

Regulatory Behaviors
    Angina
    Diaphoresis
    Hypotension
    Tachy–brady arrhythmias
    Oliguria

Cognitive Behaviors
    Apprehension
    Anxiousness
    Confusion
    Restlessness
    Altered thought process
    Nervousness

NURSING RESPONSIBILITIES

Assessment
    Assess regulatory behaviors indicative of decreased coronary
       artery perfusion (I)
    Assess cognitive behaviors indicative of decreased coronary
       artery perfusion (I)
    Monitor the side or therapeutic effects of prescribed drugs
       (I)
    Monitor the ECG pattern continuously (I)
    Auscultate the heart for abnormal heart sounds (I)

Interventions

Fluid
    Evaluate with the physician the results of specific hemo-
       dynamic parameters: coronary flow velocity, mean flow
       ml/min, and calculated mean coronary resistance mmHg/
       ml/min (D)
    Administer prescribed medications (D)

Evaluate data from hemodynamic parameters, if available: PAP, PCWP, CVP, SVR, and CO (I)

Evaluate the pulse for rate, rhythm, volume, and jugular-vein distension (I)

Measure arterial blood pressure and MAP (I)

Regulate the IV flow rate and check patency (I)

Measure and record intake, output, and specific gravity (I)

Check for the presence/absence of peripheral pulses and for bilateral equality (I)

Evaluate laboratory studies and inform the physician of any significant deviations (I)

Evaluate for the presence/absence of edema (I)

Aeration

Provide humidified oxygen via mask, nasal catheter, or nasal cannula at the prescribed flow rate (I)

Evaluate the skin color (I)

Evaluate the effectiveness of oxygen or ventilatory support (I)

Reduce extraneous environmental stimuli (I)

Nutrition

Limit dietary intake until the patient's condition stabilizes (I)

Provide gradual intake of a low-salt diet (I)

Assist the patient with the prescribed diet (I)

Communication

Listen to patient and family concerns (I)

Reduce the patient's anxiety (I)

Provide knowledge regarding diagnostic and treatment procedures (I)

Instruct the patient regarding changes in lifestyle: diet, medication, exercise, etc. (I)

Activity

Encourage positional changes that are conducive to ventricular contraction and cardiac output (I)

Limit physical activity until coronary artery perfusion dynamics stabilize and the patient is pain-free (I)

Encourage the use of diversional activities (I)

Encourage passive range-of-motion exercises (I)

Pain
    Administer analgesics as prescribed (D)
    Evaluate the type, location, and duration of pain (I)

Bibliography
Berne, R. & Levy, M. *Cardiovascular physiology.* St. Louis: C. V.
    Mosby, 1981.
Braunwald, E. & Sobel, B. Coronary blood flow and myocardial
    ischemia, in Braunwald, E. (ed.), *Heart disease: A textbook of
    cardiovascular medicine.* Philadelphia: W. B. Saunders, 1984, pp.
    1235–1261.

Peripheral Tissue Perfusion, Decreased

DEFINITION
A clinical state whereby the individual experiences, or has the
potential to experience, a decrease in nutrition and respiration
at the cellular level due to a decrease in capillary blood flow.

ETIOLOGY
    Hypovolemia
    Thrombocytosis
    Diabetes mellitus
    Congestive heart failure
    Myocardial infarction
    Coronary artery spasm
    Peripheral artery vasospasm
    Vasoconstriction
    Anemia
    Disseminated intravascular coagulation (DIC)
    Cancer or tumor
    Edema
    Septic shock
    Prolonged immobility
    Invasive procedures
    Blood vessel trauma
    Anorexia or malnutrition
    Obesity
    Trauma

DEFINING CHARACTERISTICS

Regulatory Behaviors
Cool extremities
Diminished peripheral pulsations
Pallor
Cyanosis
Claudication
Edema
Lack of lanugo hair
Loss of sensory function
Bruits
Slow-healing lesions
Slow-growing, dry, thick nails
Prickling sensation

Cognitive Behaviors
Unknown

NURSING RESPONSIBILITIES

Assessment
Assess regulatory behaviors indicative of decreased peripheral tissue perfusion (I)
Observe the side or therapeutic effects of prescribed medications (I)
Inspect the skin for color, temperature, and hydration (I)
Palpate the peripheral pulses for quality and equality (I)
Auscultate the heart for abnormal heart sounds (I)
Inspect the lower extremities for edema (I)

Interventions

Fluid
Administer prescribed medications (D)
Evaluate for cutaneous perfusion (I)
Report changes such as cool, pale, cyanotic, moist, or clammy skin (I)
Measure intake, output, and specific gravity (I)
Record daily weight (I)

Measure arterial blood pressure, peripheral blood pressure, and MAP (I)

Evaluate data from hemodynamic parameters, if available: PAP, PCWP, CVP, and CO (I)

Evaluate systemic vascular resistance (I)

Regulate the IV flow rate and check for patency (I)

Evaluate laboratory studies (I)

Use aseptic techniques when handling IV lines (I)

Aeration

Provide humidified oxygen via mask, nasal cannula, or nasal prongs at the prescribed flow rate (D)

Evaluate the patient's skin color (I)

Evaluate the effectiveness of oxygen or ventilatory support (I)

Nutrition

Assist the patient with the prescribed diet (I)

Incorporate the patient's food preferences into his or her diet, when possible (I)

Communication

Listen to the patient's concerns and fears (I)

Reduce the patient's anxiety level (I)

Provide knowledge regarding diagnostic and treatment procedures (I)

Activity

Apply antiembolic stockings (ID)

Change CVP or Swan-Ganz dressings q24h prn or according to unit protocol (I)

Help the patient to change position on a regular basis (I)

Ambulate the patient as soon as possible (I)

Pain

Instruct the patient to avoid crossing his or her legs (I)

Administer prescribed analgesics (I)

Bibliography

Berne, R. & Levy, M. *Cardiovascular physiology.* St. Louis: C. V. Mosby, 1981.

Carpenito, L. J. *Handbook of nursing diagnosis.* Philadelphia: Lippincott, 1984.

Gettrust, K., Ryan, S., & Engleman, D. *Applied nursing diagnosis.*
    New York: Wiley, 1985.
Kim, M. J., McFarland, G., & McLane, A. *Nursing diagnosis.* St. Louis:
    C. V. Mosby, 1984.

Peripheral Tissue Perfusion, Obstructed, Thrombophlebitis

DEFINITION
Thrombophlebitis denotes the presence of venous thromboses and inflammation.

ETIOLOGY
Superficial thrombophlebitis
 Inflammatory nodular lesion
  Erythema nodosum
  Erythema induration
  Periarteritis nodosa
 Deep thrombophlebitis
  Cellulitis
  Lymphedema
  Sudden arterial occlusion
  Ruptured Baker's cyst
  Injury to endothelium
   Thromboangitis obliterans
   Septic thrombophlebitis
   IV injection
   Indwelling catheters

DEFINING CHARACTERISTICS

Regulatory Behaviors
Tenderness
Redness
Induration along vein
Pain
Swelling
Cyanosis
Venous distension

Cognitive Behaviors
>   Sensation of discomfort
>   Apprehension

NURSING RESPONSIBILITIES

Assessment

>   Assess regulatory behaviors indicative of thrombophlebitis (I)
>   Assess cognitive behaviors indicative of thrombophlebitis (I)
>   Observe the side or therapeutic effects of prescribed medications (I)
>   Palpate the peripheral pulses for quality and equality (I)
>   Inspect the lower extremities for edema (I)
>   Auscultate the heart for abnormal heart sounds (I)

Interventions

Fluid

>   Administer prescribed medications (D)
>>   Heparin, 5000–10,000 units IV as constant infusion or 1000–2000 units per hour
>>   Coumadin
>>   Streptokinase
>>   Urokinase
>   Regulate the IV flow rate and check the site for any redness (I)
>   Evaluate cutaneous perfusion (I)
>   Evaluate the skin for color, temperature, and hydration (I)
>   Report changes such as cool, pale, cyanotic, moist, or clammy skin (I)
>   Measure intake, output, and specific gravity (I)
>   Evaluate systemic vascular resistance (I)
>   Evaluate data from hemodynamic parameters if available: PAP, PCWP, CVP, and CO (I)
>   Evaluate for signs of venous thrombosis: positive Homan's sign and presence of tenderness (I)
>   Compare the circumferential measurements of each calf to detect small degrees of unilateral swelling (I)
>   Evaluate partial thromboplastin time (PTT) (I)
>   Measure blood pressure and MAP (I)

Aeration
> Provide humidified oxygen via mask, nasal prongs, or nasal catheter at the prescribed flow rate (I)
> Evaluate the patient's skin color (I)
> Reduce extraneous environmental stimuli (I)

Nutrition
> Assist the patient with the prescribed diet (I)
> Incorporate the patient's food preferences into his or her diet, when possible (I)

Communication
> Assist the physician as he or she explains diagnostic procedures to the patient and family (I)
>> Doppler ultrasound
>>> Ultrasound is reflected from moving red blood cells within the vessel and is shifted in frequency by an amount proportional to the flow velocity
>> Segmental limb pressure
>>> A pressure index, or percentage of brachial pressure, is calculated by comparing the systolic pressure in the lower extremity with that of the upper extremity
> Listen to patient and family concerns (I)
> Reduce the patient's anxiety level (I)

Activity
> Encourage ambulation, when acceptable (I)
> Instruct the patient not to cross his or her legs while lying in bed (I)
> Encourage the use of diversional activities (I)
> Encourage passive range-of-motion exercises (I)

Pain
> Administer prescribed analgesics (D)
> Evaluate the type, location, and duration of pain (I)

Bibliography

Johanson, B., Dungca, C., Hoffmeister, D., & Wells, S. *Standards for critical care* (2nd ed.). St. Louis: C. V. Mosby, 1985.
Peterson, L. Perioperative vascular monitoring. *Critical Care Quarterly*, 8(2), pp. 1–9, September 1985.

CARDIOPULMONARY STABILITY, ALTERATION IN

Alteration in Cardiopulmonary Stability, Chest Injury Shock

DEFINITION
Chest injury shock, caused by injuries, is more often the result of deranged cardiorespiratory function than of blood loss.

ETIOLOGY
Closed tension pneumothorax
Tension pneumothorax
    Emphysematous blebs or bullae
Open pneumothorax
    Penetrating wounds
Rib fractures
Blunt chest trauma

DEFINING CHARACTERISTICS

Regulatory Behaviors
Cyanosis
Dyspnea
Dizziness
Decreased cardiac output
Hypotension
Tachycardia
Weakness
Pain

Cognitive Behaviors
Apprehension
Nervousness
Anxiousness
Restlessness
Fear

NURSING RESPONSIBILITIES

Assessment
Assess regulatory behaviors indicative of chest injury shock
    (I)

Assess cognitive behaviors indicative of chest injury shock (I)

Monitor the ECG pattern continuously (I)

Assess for the presence of pneumothorax (I)

Observe the side or therapeutic effects of prescribed medications (I)

Auscultate the heart for rate, rhythm, and regularity (I)

Auscultate the heart for abnormal heart sounds (I)

Palpate for the presence of peripheral pulses and check for bilateral equality (I)

Auscultate the chest for respiratory rate, rhythm, and regularity (I)

Inspect chest movement for labored breathing and symmetry (I)

Inspect the skin for cyanosis (I)

Percuss the posterior chest for decreased diaphragmatic descent (I)

Palpate the chest for a precordial leave (I)

Interventions

Fluid

Administer prescribed medications (D)

Administer prescribed IV fluids (D)

Evaluate the skin for edema, color, temperature, and diaphoresis (I)

Evaluate data from hemodynamic parameters: PAP, PCWP, CVP, CO, and SVR (I)

Measure arterial blood pressure and MAP (I)

Regulate the IV flow rate and check for patency (I)

Measure intake, urinary volume, and specific gravity (I)

Evaluate laboratory studies (I)

Aeration

Administer humidified oxygen by mask, nasal catheter, or nasal prongs at the prescribed flow rate (D)

Provide ventilatory support (ID)

Evaluate the effectiveness of the chest tube and the amount of drainage (I)

Evaluate hemoglobin, hematocrit, and arterial blood gasses (I)

Suction the patient via mouth, airway, endotracheal tube, or tracheostomy tube while using aseptic techniques (I)

Measure pulmonary vascular resistance (I)

Nutrition

Provide the patient with a prescribed low-salt diet (D)

Adjust the diet to the patient's lifestyle (ID)

Assist the patient with his or her diet (I)

Communication

Reduce the patient's anxiety level (I)

Keep teaching on a simple level, then progress to a more complex level, depending upon the patient (I)

Provide knowledge regarding diagnostic procedures or supportive devices (I)

Prepare the patient and his or her family for the possibility of surgery (I)

Activity

Immobilize the patient until the extent of the injuries can be determined (I)

Evaluate the abdomen for abnormal bowel sounds (I)

Pain

Administer analgesics as prescribed (I)

Evaluate the type, location, and duration of pain (I)

Bibliography

Borg, N., Nikas, D., Stark, J., & Williams, S. *Core curriculum for critical care nursing* (2nd ed.). Philadelphia: W. B. Saunders, 1981.

Bordicks, K. *Patterns of shock implications for nursing care* (2nd ed.). New York: Macmillan, 1980.

Alteration in Cardiopulmonary Stability, Cardiogenic Shock

DEFINITION

Shock caused by heart failure is called cardiogenic shock or cardiac shock; it leads to decreased cardiac output.

ETIOLOGY

Left myocardial infarction

Rupture of the interventricular septum

    Coronary embolus
    Rupture of aortic aneurysm
    Dissecting aortic aneurysm
    Direct trauma to the heart
    Serious cardiac arrhythmias
    Shock related to cardiac surgery
    Obstruction of venous inflow to the right atrium
    Tension pneumothorax
    Mediastinal shift
    Embolus in the vena cava
    Cardiac tamponade

DEFINING CHARACTERISTICS

Regulatory Behaviors
    Rapid and thready pulse
    Hypotension
    Decreased pulse pressure
    Distended neck veins
    Increased CVP
    Increased PCWP
    Pallor
    Cyanosis
    Peripheral edema
    Tachypnea
    Dyspnea
    Pulmonary congestion
    Oliguria

Cognitive Behaviors
    Irritability
    Anxiety
    Apathy
    Lethargy
    Confusion
    Unconsciousness

NURSING RESPONSIBILITIES

Assessment
    Assess regulatory behaviors indicative of cardiogenic shock
       (I)
    Assess cognitive behaviors indicative of cardiogenic shock (I)

Monitor the ECG pattern continuously (I)

Observe the side or therapeutic effects of prescribed medications (I)

Assess the patient's neurological status (I)

Assess the effectiveness of counterpulsation (I)

Inspect the skin for edema (I)

Auscultate the heart for rate, rhythm, and regularity (I)

Auscultate the heart for abnormal heart sounds (I)

Palpate for the presence of peripheral pulses and check for bilateral equality (I)

Palpate the chest for thrill (I)

Palpate the chest for abnormal precordial thrust (I)

Auscultate the chest for adventitious breath sounds (I)

Auscultate the chest for respiratory rate, rhythm, and regularity (I)

Palpate the chest for vocal or tactile fremitus (I)

Inspect chest movement for labored breathing and symmetry (I)

Inspect the skin for cyanosis (I)

Percuss the chest for abnormal resonance (I)

Percuss the posterior chest for decreased diaphragmatic descent (I)

Palpate the chest for a precordial heave (I)

Auscultate the abdomen for abnormal bowel sounds (I)

Interventions

Fluid

Administer prescribed IV fluids (D)

Administer prescribed medications (D)

    Dopamine

    Dobutamine

    Isoproterenol

    Norepinephrine

    Nitroprusside

    Methylprednisolone

    Lasix

    Edecrin

    Morphine sulfate

    Intravenous nitroglycerin

Evaluate the skin for color, temperature, and diaphoresis (I)

Evaluate data from hemodynamic parameters: PAP, PCWP, CVP, CO, and SVR (I)

Measure arterial blood pressure and MAP (I)

Regulate the IV flow rate and check for patency (I)

Measure intake, urinary volume, and specific gravity (I)

Evaluate the patient's weight (I)

Evaluate laboratory studies (I)

Evaluate the jugular veins for distension (I)

Aeration

Administer humidified oxygen by mask, nasal catheter, or nasal prongs at the prescribed flow rate (D)

Provide ventilatory support (ID)

Evaluate hemoglobin, hematocrit, and arterial blood gasses (I)

Suction the patient via mouth, airway, endotracheal tube, or tracheostomy tube while using aseptic technique (I)

Instruct the patient to cough, turn, and deep breathe (I)

Measure pulmonary vascular resistance (I)

Nutrition

Provide the patient with a prescribed low-salt diet (D)

Adjust the diet to the patient's lifestyle (ID)

Assist the patient with the diet (I)

Communication

Reduce the patient's anxiety level (I)

Arrange situations that encourage the patient's autonomy (I)

Keep teaching on a simple level, then progress to more complex levels, depending upon the patient (I)

Provide knowledge regarding diagnostic procedures or supportive devices (I)

Inform the physician of any changes in the patient's condition (I)

Listen to the patient's concerns, fears, and anxieties (I)

Activity

Provide counterpulsation to decrease afterload and increase coronary artery perfusion (D)

Change the patient's position q2h (I)

Elevate the head of the bed (I)

Provide rest and moderate activity periods (I)

Apply antiembolic support stockings (I)

Encourage the use of diversional activities (I)

Apply appropriate antiseptic around the IV tubing connections to prevent infection (I)

Pain

Administer analgesics as prescribed (I)

Evaluate the type, location, and duration of pain (I)

Ask the patient what makes him or her feel comfortable (I)

Bibliography

Bordicks, K. *Patterns of shock implications for nursing care* (2nd ed.). New York: Macmillan, 1980.

Borg, N., Nikas, D., Stark, J., & Williams, S. *Core curriculum for critical care nursing* (2nd ed.). Philadelphia: W. B. Saunders, 1981.

TISSUE PERFUSION, ALTERATION IN

Vasodilatation of Vascular Bed, Anaphylactic Shock

DEFINITION

Anaphylactic shock is an allergic or hypersensitivity reaction causing marked loss of plasma from the vascular compartment into the interstitial compartment.

ETIOLOGY

Hypersensitivity to medications

Curare

Mannitol

Acetylsalicylic acid

Aminopyrine

Indomethacin

Radiopaque contrast material

Penicillins

Cephalosporins

Tetracyclines

Amphotericin B

Nitrofurantoin

Aminoglycosides

Lidocaine

Procaine

Pollens
Foods
  Eggs
  Seafood
  Nuts
  Grains
  Beans
  Cottonseed oil
  Chocolate
  Poultry

DEFINING CHARACTERISTICS

Regulatory Behaviors
Decreased cardiac output
Hypotension
Dizziness
Dyspnea
Cyanosis
Edema
Itching
Diffuse erythema
Abdominal cramps
Vomiting
Diarrhea
Arrhythmias

Cognitive Behaviors
Anxiety
Nervousness
Apprehension
Restlessness
Unconsciousness

NURSING RESPONSIBILITIES

Assessment
Assess regulatory behaviors indicative of anaphylactic shock
(I)
Assess cognitive behaviors indicative of anaphylactic shock
(I)
Assess the patient's medical history for possible allergies (I)

Observe the side or therapeutic effects of prescribed medications (I)

Auscultate the heart for abnormal heart sounds (I)

Auscultate the heart for rate, rhythm, and regularity (I)

Inspect for dyspnea (I)

Auscultate the chest for adventitious breath sounds (I)

Auscultate the chest for respiratory rate, rhythm, and regularity (I)

Intervention

Fluid

Administer prescribed medications (D)

    Epinephrine

Check for the presence/absence of peripheral pulses and for bilateral equality (I)

Measure arterial blood pressure and MAP (I)

Administer appropriate IV fluids (I)

Regulate the IV flow rate and check for patency (I)

Evaluate data from hemodynamic parameters: PAP, PCWP, CVP, SVR, and CO (I)

Measure intake and output (I)

Evaluate the skin for color, temperature, and diaphoresis (I)

Evaluate laboratory studies (I)

Aeration

Establish and maintain a patent airway via endotracheal tube or tracheostomy (D)

Maintain adequate ventilation through the use of continuous ventilatory support (D)

Administer humidified oxygen by mask, nasal prongs, or nasal catheter at the prescribed flow rate (I)

Obtain arterial blood gasses from an arterial line (I)

Nutrition

Encourage the patient to maintain the prescribed diet (I)

Assist the patient with eating (I)

Evaluate which foods cause an allergic reaction (I)

Consult with the dietitian (I)

Communication

Reduce the patient's anxiety level (I)

Inform the physician of any changes in the patient's condition (I)

Provide knowledge regarding the causes of anaphylactic shock (I)

Activity
Change the patient's position q2h (I)
Encourage alternative rest and moderate activity periods (I)

Pain
Discuss possible pain-relieving measures (I)
Evaluate the type, location, and duration of pain (I)

Bibliography
Bordick, K. *Patterns of shock implications for nursing care* (2nd. ed.), New York: Macmillan, 1980.

CARDIAC RHYTHM, ALTERATION IN

Sinus Conduction Alteration, Sinus Arrhythmias

DEFINITION
Sinus arrhythmia is characterized by a phasic variation in cycle length of greater than 0.16 seconds during sinus rhythm.

ETIOLOGY
Aged, with slower heart rate
Enhanced vagal tone
Digitalis
Morphine

DEFINING CHARACTERISTICS

Regulatory Behaviors
Palpitations
Dizziness
Syncope

Cognitive Behaviors
None

NURSING RESPONSIBILITIES

Assessment

Assess regulatory behaviors indicative of sinus arrhythmias (I)

Assess the respiratory form of sinus arrhythmia in which the P–P interval cyclically shortens during inspiration (I)

Observe the side or therapeutic effects of prescribed medications (I)

Intervention

Fluid

Administer prescribed medications (D)
  Sedatives
  Tranquilizers
  Atropine
  Ephedrine
  Isoproterenol

Regulate the IV flow rate (I)

Measure the apical rate and rhythm (I)

Measure the components of ECG reflecting sinus arrhythmia (I)

> P wave: precede each QRS with normal, fairly constant contour
> P–R interval: normal, constant (0.12 sec)
> QRS: normal (0.08 sec)

Measure blood pressure (I)

Aeration

Provide oxygen via mask, nasal catheter, or nasal prongs at the prescribed flow rate (D)

Nutrition

Encourage the patient to eat a low-salt diet (I)

Communication

Provide knowledge regarding possible causes of sinus arrhythmias (I)

Listen to the patient's verbalization of concerns, fears, and anxieties (I)

Reduce the patient's anxiety level (I)

Activity
Provide physical activity to increase the heart rate (ID)

Pain
Provide comfort measures for any discomfort experienced by the patient (I)

Bibliography

Andreoli, K., Fowkes, V., Zipes, D., & Wallace, A. *Comprehensive cardiac care.* St. Louis: C. V. Mosby, 1979.

Sinus Conduction Alteration, Sinus Tachycardia

DEFINITION
Sinus tachycardia is present when the heart beat is regular and the rate is between 100 and 150 bpm.

ETIOLOGY
Fever
Hypotension
Thyrotoxicosis
Anemia
Anxiety
Exertion
Hypovolemia
Pulmonary emboli
Myocardial infarction
Congestive heart failure
Shock
Pericarditis
Medications
Atropine
Bronchodilators
Epinephrine
Nicotine
Caffeine

DEFINING CHARACTERISTICS

Regulatory Behaviors
Angina
Dyspnea

Shortness of breath
Cool extremities
Oliguria

Cognitive Behaviors
Anxiousness
Restlessness
Expression of discomfort

NURSING RESPONSIBILITIES

Assessment

Assess regulatory behaviors indicative of sinus tachycardia (I)

Assess cognitive behaviors indicative of sinus tachycardia (I)

Observe the side and therapeutic effects of prescribed medications (I)

Auscultate the chest for respiratory rate, rhythm, and regularity (I)

Auscultate the chest for adventitious breath sounds (I)

Interventions

Fluid

Administer prescribed medications (D)
Propranolol
Verapamil (Isoptin)

Measure the apical rate and rhythm (I)

Measure the components of ECG reflecting sinus tachycardia (I)

P wave: normal contour, but can develop a larger amplitude and become peaked

P–P interval: varies slightly from cycle to cycle

P–R interval: shortened

Regulate the IV flow rate (I)

Measure blood pressure and other factors reflecting hemodynamic stability/instability (I)

Aeration

Maintain oxygenation via mask, nasal cannula, or nasal catheter at the flow rate prescribed by the physician (D)

Provide a position comfortable for O_2–CO_2 exchange (I)

Nutrition
    Eliminate stimulants from the patient's diet (I)
        Tobacco
        Caffeine
        Alcohol
    Encourage the patient to maintain a low-salt diet (I)
    Assist the patient with eating if necessary (I)
    Provide a spiritual support system (I)

Communication
    Reduce the patient's anxiety level (I)
    Encourage the patient to verbalize his or her fears, anxieties, and concerns (I)
    Provide knowledge regarding the causes of sinus tachycardia (I)
    Provide knowledge regarding the need for diagnostic procedures and supportive devices (I)

Activity
    Provide adequate rest periods (I)
    Reduce physical activity until tachycardia has subsided (I)
    Provide diversional activities (I)

Pain
    Administer analgesics to relieve pain (D)
    Teach the patient stress-reduction techniques (I)

Bibliography

Andreoli, K., Fowkes, V., Zipes, D., & Wallace, A. *Comprehensive cardiac care.* St. Louis: C. V. Mosby, 1979.

Sinus Conduction Alteration, Sinus Bradycardia

DEFINITION
Sinus bradycardia exists when the sinus node discharges at a rate of less than 60 bpm.

ETIOLOGY
    Excessive vagal or decreased sympathetic tone
    Eye surgery
    Meningitis

Intracranial tumor
Cervical tumor
Mediastinal tumor
Inferior myocardial infarction
Myxedema
Obstructive jaundice
Cardiac fibrosis
Vasovagal syncope
Carotid sinus stimulation
Vomiting
Hypothermia
Medications
    Propranolol
    Neostigmine
    Clonidine
    Calcium channel blockers
    Digitalis

DEFINING CHARACTERISTICS

Regulatory Behaviors
Weakness
Faintness
Salivation
Palpitations
Dizziness
Syncope

Cognitive Behaviors
Nervousness
Anxiousness
Fearfulness

NURSING RESPONSIBILITIES

Assessment
Assess regulatory behaviors indicative of sinus bradycardia (I)

Assess cognitive behaviors indicative of sinus bradycardia (I)

Observe the side and therapeutic effects of prescribed medications (I)

Assess the effectiveness of pacemaker function, if required to treat sinus bradycardia (I)

Auscultate the heart for abnormal heart sounds (I)
Auscultate the heart for apical heart rate and rhythm (I)
Auscultate the chest for adventitious breath sounds (I)
Auscultate the chest for respiratory rate, rhythm, and regularity (I)

Intervention

Fluid

Administer prescribed medications (D)

    Atropine
    Isoproterenol
    Ephedrine
    Epinephrine
    Hydralazine

Measure blood pressure and MAP (I)

Evaluate data from hemodynamic parameters, if available: PAP, PCWP, CVP, SVR, and CO (I)

Measure the components of ECG reflecting sinus bradycardia (I)

    P wave: normal contour
    P–R interval: greater than 0.12 sec
    QRS: normal, with P wave preceding each QRS

Regulate the IV flow rate (I)

Aeration

Provide oxygenation via mask, nasal catheter, or nasal prongs at the flow rate prescribed by the physician (D)

Nutrition

Encourage the patient to maintain the prescribed diet (I)
Provide an atmosphere conducive to eating (I)
Provide a spiritual support system (I)

Communication

Reduce meaningless environmental stimuli so that the patient can rest and sleep (I)
Instruct the patient regarding the critical care environment and the need for diagnostic or supportive devices (I)
Reduce the patient's anxiety level (I)
Notify the physician of any changes in pacemaker function (I)

Activity
    Assist the physician with temporary pacemaker insertion
        and/or regulation (I)
    Encourage physical activity, when realistic (I)

Pain
    Administer analgesics as prescribed for discomfort (D)
    Provide comfort measures (I)

Bibliography

Andreoli, K., Fowkes, V., Zipes, D., & Wallace, A. *Comprehensive
    cardiac care.* St. Louis: C. V. Mosby, 1979.
Davis, D. *How to quickly and accurately master EKG interpretation.*
    Philadelphia: Lippincott, 1985.

Sinus Conduction Alteration,
Sinus Pause or Block

DEFINITION
In sinus arrest or pause, there is an absence of atrial depolarization; periods of ventricular systole result if escape beats produced by latent pacemakers do not discharge.

ETIOLOGY
    Acute myocardial infarction
    Degenerative fibrotic changes
    Digitalis intoxication

DEFINING CHARACTERISTICS

Regulatory Behaviors
    Slow heart rate
    Weakness
    Faintness
    Palpitation
    Dizziness
    Syncope

Cognitive Behaviors
    Nervousness
    Anxiousness
    Apprehension

NURSING RESPONSIBILITIES

Assessment

 Assess regulatory behaviors indicative of sinus pause or block (I)

 Assess cognitive behaviors indicative of sinus pause or block (I)

 Monitor the side or therapeutic effects of prescribed medications (I)

 Auscultate the heart for abnormal heart sounds (I)

 Auscultate the heart for apical heart rate and rhythm (I)

 Auscultate the chest for adventitious breath sounds (I)

 Auscultate the chest for respiratory rate, rhythm, and regularity (I)

Interventions

Fluid

 Administer prescribed medications (D)

  Atropine 0.4–0.5 mg to a maximum of 2 mg

  Isuprel 2–4 μg/min and increase gradually

 Measure blood pressure and MAP (I)

 Evaluate data from hemodynamic parameters: PAP, PCWP, CVP, SVR, and CO (I)

 Measure the components of ECG reflecting sinus pause or block (I)

  Sinus pause

   P–P interval delimiting, and pause does not equal a multiple of the basic interval

   R–R varies due to the pause

  Sinus arrest

   Absent PQRST

 Regulate the IV flow rate (I)

Aeration

Provide humidified oxygen via mask, nasal catheter, or nasal prongs at the prescribed flow rate (D)

Nutrition

 Encourage the patient to eat the prescribed diet (I)

 Provide an atmosphere conducive to eating (I)

Communication
> Reduce meaningless environmental stimuli so that the patient can rest and sleep (I)
>
> Reduce the patient's anxiety level (I)

Activity
> Assist the physician with temporary pacemaker insertion and/or regulation (I)
>
> Encourage physical activity, when realistic (I)

Pain
> Administer analgesics as prescribed for discomfort (D)
>
> Provide comfort measures (I)

Bibliography

Andreoli, K., Fowkes, V., Zipes, D., & Wallace, A. *Comprehensive cardiac care*. St. Louis: C. V. Mosby, 1979.

Shepard, N., Vaughan, P., & Rice, V. A guide to arrhythmia interpretation and management. *Critical Care Nurse*, 58-85, September-October 1982.

Zipes, D. Specific arrhythmias: Diagnosis and treatment, in Braunwald, E. (ed.), *Heart disease: a textbook of cardiovascular medicine*. Philadelphia: W. B. Saunders, 1984, pp. 683-743.

Sinus Conduction Alteration, Sinoatrial (S-A) Exit Block

DEFINITION

Sinoatrial (S-A) block is a conductive disturbance during which an impulse formed within the S-A node is blocked from depolarizing the atria.

ETIOLOGY

> Excessive vagal stimulation
>
> Acute myocarditis
>
> Myocardial infarction
>
> Myocardial fibrosis
>
> Medications
>> Quinidine
>>
>> Procainamide
>>
>> Digitalis

Acute infections
  Diphtheria
  Rheumatic carditis
Atherosclerosis

DEFINING CHARACTERISTICS

Regulatory Behaviors
Weakness
Faintness
Palpitations
Dizziness
Syncope

Cognitive Behaviors
Nervousness
Anxiousness
Apprehension

NURSING RESPONSIBILITIES

Assessment
Assess regulatory behaviors indicative of S–A exit block (I)
Assess cognitive behaviors indicative of S–A exit block (I)
Monitor the side or therapeutic effects of prescribed medications (I)
Assess the functioning and effectiveness of atrial or ventricular pacing (I)
Auscultate the chest for adventitious breath sounds (I)

Interventions

Fluid
Administer prescribed medications (D)
  Atropine
  Isoproterenol
Administer the prescribed IV fluids (D)
Measure the components of ECG reflecting S–A exit block (I)
  P-wave: absent; producing a pause; duration of which is a multiple of the basic P–P interval
  QRS: absent
Measure blood pressure and MAP (I)
Measure intake and urinary volume (I)

Aeration

Provide humidified oxygen via mask, nasal catheter, or nasal cannula at the prescribed flow rate (D)

Nutrition

Provide a spiritual support system (I)

Encourage the patient to maintain the prescribed diet (I)

Communication

Reduce the patient's anxiety level (I)

Notify the physician of any changes in pacemaker function (I)

Activity

Encourage physical activity, when realistic (I)

Pain

Administer prescribed analgesics (D)

Evaluate the type, location, and duration of pain (I)

Bibliography

Andreoli, K., Fowkes, V., Zipes, D., & Wallace, A. *Comprehensive cardiac care*. St. Louis: C. V. Mosby, 1979.

Shephard, N., Vaughan, P., & Rice, V. A guide to arrhythmia interpretation and management. *Critical Care Nurse*, 58-85, September-October 1982.

Zipes, D. Specific arrhythmias: Diagnosis and treatment in Braunwald, E. (ed.), *Heart disease: A textbook of cardiovascular medicine*. Philadelphia: W. B. Saunders, 1984, pp. 683-743.

Atrial Conduction Alteration, Premature Atrial Contraction

DEFINITION

Premature atrial beats originate in the atria from pacemaker cells located outside the S-A node.

ETIOLOGY

Infection

Inflammation

Myocardial ischemia

Medication

Digitalis

Tension
Tobacco
Caffeine
Hypoxia
Gastrointestinal disease

DEFINING CHARACTERISTICS

Regulatory Behaviors
Palpitations
Weakness
Fatigue
Recurrent tachycardias

Cognitive Behaviors
Anxiousness
Nervousness
Apprehension

NURSING RESPONSIBILITIES

Assessment
Assess regulatory behaviors indicative of premature atrial contractions (I)
Assess cognitive behaviors indicative of premature atrial contractions (I)
Observe the side or therapeutic effects of prescribed medications (I)
Auscultate the heart for abnormal heart sounds (I)
Auscultate the heart for apical heart rate and rhythm (I)
Auscultate the chest for adventitious breath sounds (I)
Auscultate the chest for respiratory rate, rhythm, and regularity (I)

Interventions

Fluid
Administer prescribed medications (D)
Digitalis
Quinidine
Procainamide
Measure blood pressure and MAP (I)
Evaluate data from hemodynamic parameters: PAP, PCWP, CVP, SVR, and CO (I)

Regulate the IV flow rate (I)

Measure the components of ECG reflecting premature atrial
   contraction (I)
   P wave: early, abnormal
   QRS: present or absent
   P-R interval: different from dominant P-R; 0.12 sec
      or greater
   Compensatory pause: incomplete (beat interrupts or
      resets the basic rhythm)

Aeration

Provide humidified oxygenation by mask, nasal catheter, or
   nasal prongs at the prescribed flow rate (D)

Nutrition

Encourage the patient to maintain the prescribed diet (I)
Provide an atmosphere conducive to eating (I)
Provide a spiritual support system (I)

Communication

Reduce meaningless environmental stimuli so that the
   patient can rest or sleep (I)
Reduce the patient's anxiety level (I)
Notify the physician of any changes in the patient's condition (I)

Activity

Encourage physical activity (I)
Encourage patient participation in self-care (I)

Pain

Provide necessary comfort measures (I)

Bibliography

Andreoli, K., Fowkes, V., Zipes, D., & Wallace, A. *Comprehensive
   cardiac care.* St. Louis: C. V. Mosby, 1979.

Shepard, N., Vaughan, P., & Rice, V. A guide to arrhythmia interpretation and management. *Critical Care Nurse*, 1092, 58–85, September-
   October 1982.

Zipes, D. Specific arrhythmias: Diagnosis and treatment in Braunwald,
   E. (ed.), *Heart disease: A textbook of cardiovascular medicine.*
   Philadelphia: W. B. Saunders, 1984, pp. 683–743.

Atrial Conduction Alteration, Paroxysmal Atrial Tachycardia

DEFINITION

Paroxysmal atrial tachycardia (PAT) is characterized by a rapid, regular, atrial tachycardia of sudden onset and termination, occurring at rates generally between 150 and 250 bpm.

ETIOLOGY

Coronary artery disease
Thyrotoxicosis
Overexcitation
Emotional stimuli
Caffeine
Nicotine

DEFINING CHARACTERISTICS

Regulatory Behaviors
Palpitations
Angina
Heart failure
Shock
Syncope
Decreased cardiac output
Decreased stroke volume
Fatigue

Cognitive Behaviors
Nervousness
Anxiety
Apprehension

NURSING RESPONSIBILITIES

Assessment
Assess regulatory behaviors indicative of PAT (I)
Assess cognitive behaviors indicative of PAT (I)
Monitor situations in which PAT occurs (I)
Assess both prehospital experience with PAT and coping mechanisms used during PAT episodes (I)
Assess the neck veins for distension (I)

Auscultate the heart for abnormal heart sounds (I)
Auscultate the heart for rate and rhythm (I)
Auscultate the chest for adventitious heart sounds (I)

Interventions

Fluid

Administer prescribed medications (D)
Vasoconstrictors
    Tensilon
    Neosynephrine
    Aramine
Antiarrhythmias
    Quinidine
    Pronestyl
    Inderal
    Digitalis
Evaluate laboratory studies (D)
Measure blood pressure and MAP (I)
Obtain data from hemodynamic parameters: PAP, PCWP, CVP, and CO (I)
Measure intake and output (I)
Measure the components of ECG reflecting PAT (I)
    Atrial rate: 150–250 bpm
    P–P interval: regular
    R–R interval: regular or irregular
    P–R interval: 0.12 sec or greater
    QRS complex: normal
Regulate the IV flow rate and check for patency (I)
Interpret laboratory values (I)

Aeration

Provide oxygen via nasal cannula, nasal prongs, or mask at the prescribed flow rate (I)
Determine whether or not the oxygen flow rate is sufficient for the patient (I)
Reduce meaningless environmental stimuli (I)

Nutrition

Encourage the patient to maintain the prescribed diet (I)
Assist the patient with his or her diet, if necessary (I)
Provide a spiritual support system, if requested (I)
Recommend the elimination of caffeine from the diet (I)

Communication

Listen to the patient's fears while experiencing PAT (I)

Reassure the patient during a PAT episode (I)

Inform the physician when PAT occurs, describing the situation (I)

Provide knowledge regarding the causes of PAT (I)

Recommend that the patient stop smoking (I)

Activity

Assist the physician with cardioversion (D)

Assist the physician with carotid sinus massage (D)

Instruct the patient in how to perform the Valsalva maneuver by holding his or her breath and bearing down, if instructed by the physician (ID)

Reduce exercise until PAT ceases (I)

Pain

Administer prescribed medications (D)

Determine the type, location, and duration of pain (I)

Bibliography

Andreoli, K., Fowkes, V., Zipes, D., & Wallace, A. *Comprehensive cardiac care.* St. Louis: C. V. Mosby, 1979.

Shepard, N., Vaughan, P., & Rice, V. A guide to arrhythmia interpretation and management. *Critical Care Nurse*, 58–85, September–October, 1982.

Zipes, D. Specific arrhythmias: Diagnosis and treatment in Braunwald, E. (ed.), *Heart disease: A textbook of cardiovascular medicine.* Philadelphia: W. B. Saunders, 1984, pp. 683–743.

Atrial Conduction Alteration, Atrial Flutter

DEFINITION

Atrial flutter indicates an atrial rate of 250–350 bpm.

ETIOLOGY

Rheumatic heart disease

Ischemic heart disease

Cardiomyopathy

Caffeine

Hypoxia

Acidosis

Trauma
Septal defects
Pulmonary emboli
Mitral valve stenosis or regurgitation
Tricuspid valve stenosis or regurgitation
Chronic ventricular failure
Thyrotoxicosis
Alcoholism
Pericarditis
Fatigue

DEFINING CHARACTERISTICS

Regulatory Behaviors
Palpitation
Fatigue
Syncope
Dyspnea
Angina
Decreased cardiac output
Decreased stroke volume

Cognitive Behaviors
Anxiousness
Nervousness
Apprehension
Fatigue

NURSING RESPONSIBILITIES

Assessment
Assess regulatory behaviors indicative of atrial flutter (I)
Assess cognitive behaviors indicative of atrial flutter (I)
Assess the side and therapeutic effects of prescribed medications (I)
Auscultate the heart for abnormal breath sounds (I)
Auscultate the heart for rate and rhythm (I)
Auscultate the chest for adventitious breath sounds (I)
Auscultate the chest for rate, rhythm, and regularity (I)

Interventions

Fluid

Administer prescribed medications (D)
    Digitalis
    Quinidine
    Pronestyl
    Inderal
    Verapamil
    Tensilon
Obtain the necessary laboratory studies (D)
Measure blood pressure and MAP (I)
Evaluate data from hemodynamic parameters: PAP, PCWP,
    CVP, and CO (I)
Measure intake and output (I)
Measure the components of ECG reflecting atrial flutter (I)
    Atrial rate: 250–350 bpm
    P-P (F-F) interval: regular
    R-F interval: regular or irregular
    Baseline has saw-tooth appearance
Regulate the IV flow rate (I)
Interpret laboratory results (I)

Aeration

Provide oxygen via mask, nasal catheter, or nasal prongs at
    the prescribed flow rate (I)
Evaluate the skin color for alterations indicating insufficient
    oxygenation (I)
Reduce meaningless environmental stimuli (I)

Nutrition

Encourage the patient to maintain the prescribed low-salt
    diet (I)
Instruct both patient and family regarding the need for
    dietary change (I)
Encourage the elimination of caffeine from the diet (I)

Communication

Reduce the patient's anxiety level (I)

Provide knowledge regarding the purpose of cardioversion (I)

Obtain informed signed consent for cardioversion (I)

Recommend that the patient stop smoking (I)

Listen to the patient's concerns while experiencing atrial flutter (I)

Activity

Assist the physician with cardioversion (D)

Limit physical activity until atrial rhythm stabilizes (I)

Provide diversional activities (I)

Pain

Administer prescribed analgesics (I)

Determine the location, type, and duration of pain (I)

Bibliography

Andreoli, K., Fowkes, V., Zipes, D., & Wallace, A. *Comprehensive cardiac care.* St. Louis: C. V. Mosby, 1979.

Shepard, N., Vaughan, P., & Rice, V. A guide to arrhythmia interpretation and management. *Critical Care Nurse*, 58–85, September–October 1982.

Zipes, D. Specific arrhythmias: Diagnosis and treatment, in Braunwald, E. (ed.), *Heart disease: A textbook of cardiovascular medicine.* Philadelphia: W. B. Saunders, 1984, pp. 683–743.

Atrial Conduction Altered, Atrial Fibrillation

DEFINITION

Atrial fibrillation is characterized by a total disorganization of atrial activity without effective atrial contraction.

ETIOLOGY

Rheumatic heart disease

Mitral valve stenosis or regurgitation

Cardiomyopathy

Hypertensive heart disease

Pulmonary emboli

Pericarditis

Coronary heart disease

Thyrotoxicosis
Caffeine
Tobacco
Diabetic coma
Medications
    Catecholamines
    Ether
    Salicylates

DEFINING CHARACTERISTICS

Regulatory Behaviors
Palpitation
Dyspnea
Decreased cardiac output
S_1 variable intensity
Fatigue
Cool extremities
Angina
Cyanosis
Syncope

Cognitive Behaviors
Alteration in mental status
Anxiousness
Apprehension

NURSING RESPONSIBILITIES

Assessment
Assess regulatory behaviors indicative of atrial fibrillation (I)
Assess cognitive behaviors indicative of atrial fibrillation (I)
Observe the side and therapeutic effects of prescribed medications (I)
Assess any complications, stroke, and pulmonary emboli associated with chronic atrial fibrillation (I)
Assess the effectiveness of cardioversion (I)
Auscultate the heart for abnormal heart sounds (I)
Auscultate the heart for rate, rhythm, and regularity (I)
Inspect peripheral skin color for mottling or cyanosis, reflecting a perfusion deficit (I)
Auscultate the chest for adventitious breath sounds (I)

Auscultate the chest for respiratory rate, rhythm, and regularity (I)

Interventions

Fluid

Administer prescribed medications (D)
  Digitalis
  Quinidine
  Pronestyl
  Inderal
  Verapamil
Measure blood pressure and MAP (I)
Record intake, output, specific gravity, and color of urine (I)
Measure data from hemodynamic parameters: PAP, PCWP, CVP, and CO (I)
Evaluate the peripheral pulses for quality and equality (I)
Regulate the IV flow rate (I)
Measure the components of ECG reflecting atrial fibrillation (I)
    R–R interval: irregular
    P waves: unidentifiable

Aeration

Provide oxygenation via mask, nasal catheter, or nasal prongs at the prescribed flow rate (D)
Reduce excessive environmental stimuli (I)

Nutrition

Encourage the patient to maintain the prescribed low-salt diet (I)
Instruct the patient to eliminate caffeine from his or her diet (I)
Provide a spiritual support system (I)

Communication

Instruct the patient regarding cardioversion (ID)
Provide knowledge regarding the causes of atrial fibrillation (I)
Reduce the patient's anxiety level (I)
Listen to both patient and family expression of concerns, fears, and anxieties (I)

Instruct the patient regarding home care, including diet, medications, and activity (I)

Activity
Assist the physician with cardioversion (D)
Reduce physical activity until rhythm stabilizes, or make a decision as to when activity is appropriate (I)
Evaluate for changes in central nervous system (CNS) activity reflecting possible embolic stroke (I)
Encourage patient participation in self-care (I)

Pain
Determine the type, location, and duration of pain (I)
Administer analgesics as ordered (D)
Reduce physical discomfort with diversional activities (I)

Bibliography

Andreoli, K., Fowkes, V., Zipes, D., & Wallace, A. *Comprehensive cardiac care.* St. Louis: C. V. Mosby, 1979.

Shepard, N., Vaughan, P., & Rice, V. A guide to arrhythmia interpretation and management. *Critical Care Nurse,* 58–85, September–October 1982.

Zipes, D. Specific arrhythmias: Diagnosis and treatment in Braunwald, E. (ed.), *Heart disease: A textbook of cardiovascular medicine.* Philadelphia: W. B. Saunders, 1984, pp. 683–743.

Atrial-Ventricular Conduction Alteration, Premature Junctional Systole

DEFINITION
Premature junctional impulse or junctional extrasystole arises from excitable foci in the A–V junctional tissues.

ETIOLOGY
Rheumatic heart disease
Coronary artery disease
    Right coronary artery

DEFINING CHARACTERISTICS

Regulatory Behaviors
Palpitation

Decreased cardiac output from frequent premature junctional beat (PJB)

Cognitive Behaviors
Anxiety
Apprehension

NURSING RESPONSIBILITIES

Assessment
Assess regulatory behaviors indicative of PJB (I)
Assess cognitive behaviors indicative of PJB (I)
Monitor the ECG pattern continuously (I)
Inspect the lower extremities for color, warmth, and pulses (I)
Auscultate the heart for abnormal heart sounds (I)

Interventions

Fluid
Administer prescribed medications (D)
Digitalis
Propranolol
Evaluate the patient's hemodynamic parameters if available: PAP, PCWP, CVP, and CO (I)
Evaluate circulatory pressure and volume through vital signs (I)
Measure intake, output, and specific gravity (I)
Measure the ECG components reflecting PJB (I)
P wave of early beat can be:
in front of QRS complex with a P-R interval of less than 0.12 sec
after the QRS complex
in the QRS complex
QRS complex: early, normal
Compensatory pause: complete or incomplete
Regulate the IV flow rate (I)

Aeration
Administer humidifed oxygen via mask, nasal catheter, or nasal prongs at the prescribed flow rate (D)
Provide an environment conducive to rest and sleep (I)
Encourage the patient to rest between nursing activities (I)

Nutrition
>   Encourage the patient to maintain the prescribed diet (I)
>   Determine those patient's food preferences that comply
>   with his or her dietary restrictions (I)
>   Provide a spiritual support system (I)
>   Provide effective oral hygiene (I)

Communication
>   Provide knowledge regarding diagnostic treatment and/or
>   supportive devices (I)
>   Listen to the patient's concerns (I)
>   Reduce the patient's anxiety level (I)

Activity
>   Encourage passive and active range-of-motion exercises (I)
>   Position the patient to maintain comfort and support (I)
>   Assist the patient with planned levels of increased activity
>   (I)
>   Provide diversional activity (1)

Pain
>   Administer analgesics to relieve any discomfort (D)

Bibliography

Andreoli, K., Fowkes, V., Zipes, D., & Wallace, A. *Comprehensive cardiac care.* St. Louis: C. V. Mosby, 1979.

Sanderson, R. & Kurth, C. *The cardiac patient* (2nd. ed.). Philadelphia: W. B. Saunders, 1983.

Shepard, N., Vaughan, P., & Rice, V. A guide to arrhythmia interpretation and management. *Critical Care Nurse*, 58–85, September–October 1982.

Zipes, D. Specific arrhythmias: Diagnosis and treatment in Braunwald, E. (ed.), *Heart disease: A textbook of cardiovascular medicine.* Philadelphia: W. B. Saunders, 1984, pp. 683–743.

Atrial-Ventricular Conduction Alteration, Junctional Tachycardia

DEFINITION
Three or more consecutive and rapid A–V junctional impulses constitute junctional tachycardia.

ETIOLOGY

Inferior wall infarction
Acute rheumatic myocarditis
Coronary artery bypass surgery
Digitalis toxicity

DEFINING CHARACTERISTICS

Regulatory Behaviors

Decreased cardiac output, depending upon ventricular
response

Angina
Syncope
Weakness
Fatigue
Constant or varying S_1
Cannon a-waves in jugular venous pulse

Cognitive Behaviors

Anxiety
Apprehension
Nervousness

NURSING RESPONSIBILITIES

Assessment

Assess regulatory behaviors indicative of junctional tachy-
cardia (I)
Assess cognitive behaviors indicative of junctional tachy-
cardia (I)
Monitor the ECG pattern continuously (I)
Auscultate the heart for abnormal heart sounds (I)

Interventions

Fluid

Administer prescribed medications (D)
Pronestyl
Quinidine
Inderal
Digitalis
Evaluate jugular venous pulse (I)
Measure the ECG components reflecting junctional tachy-

cardia (I)

> P wave can be:
>> in front of the QRS complex with a P-R interval less than 0.12 sec
>> after the QRS complex
>> in the QRS complex
> R–R interval: regular
> QRS width: usually normal
> Ventricular rate: greater than 100 bpm

Evaluate the patient's hemodynamic parameters: PAP, PCWP, CVP, and CO (I)

Evaluate the patient's vital signs (I)

Measure intake, urinary volume, and specific gravity (I)

Regulate the IV flow rate (I)

Aeration

Administer humidified oxygen via mask, nasal cannula, or nasal prongs at the prescribed flow rate (D)

Provide an environment conducive to rest and sleep (I)

Encourage the patient to rest between nursing activities (I)

Nutrition

Encourage the patient to maintain the prescribed diet (I)

Determine those patient's food preferences that comply with his or her dietary restrictions (I)

Provide a spiritual support system (I)

Communication

Provide knowledge regarding diagnostic treatments and/or supportive devices (I)

Listen to the patient's concerns (I)

Reduce the patient's anxiety level (I)

Activity

Encourage passive and active range-of-motion exercises (I)

Position the patient to maintain comfort and support (I)

Assist the patient with planned levels of increased activity (I)

Provide diversional activities (I)

Pain

Administer analgesics to relieve any discomfort (I)

Bibliography

Andreoli, K., Fowkes, V., Zipes, D., & Wallace, A. *Comprehensive cardiac care*. St. Louis: C. V. Mosby, 1979.

Shepard, N., Vaughan, P., & Rice, V. A guide to arrhythmia interpretation and management. *Critical Care Nurse*, 58–85, September–October 1982.

Zipes, D. Specific arrhythmias: Diagnosis and treatment in Braunwald, E. (ed.), *Heart disease: A textbook of cardiovascular medicine*. Philadelphia: W. B. Saunders, 1984, 683–743.

Atrial–Ventricular Conduction Alteration, First Degree Block

DEFINITION

An atrio–ventricular (A–V) block occurs when impulses originating in or above the A–V node are delayed or obstructed in their passage to the ventricles.

ETIOLOGY

Rheumatic myocarditis
Coronary artery disease
A–V node degeneration
Medications
    Digitalis
    Beta blockers
    Calcium antagonist
    Quinidine
    Procainamide
    Potassium chloride
Coronary artery bypass graft
Acute myocardial infarction
Infections
    Diphtheria
    Pneumonia
    Scarlet fever
    Measles
    Mumps
    Syphilis
    Bacterial endocarditis
    Lenegre's disease
    Lev's disease

DEFINING CHARACTERISTICS

Regulatory Behaviors
S_1 diminished in intensity
A wave in jugular venous pulse

Cognitive Behaviors
Unknown

NURSING RESPONSIBILITIES

Assessment
Assess regulatory behaviors indicative of a first-degree block
(I)
Monitor the ECG pattern continuously (I)
Assess the side and therapeutic effects of prescribed medi-
cations (I)
Inspect the lower extremities for color, warmth, and pulse
(I)
Auscultate the heart for abnormal heart sounds (I)

Interventions

Fluid
Administer prescribed medications (D)
    Atropine
    Isoproterenol
Measure the ECG components reflecting a first-degree block
(I)
    Every P wave is followed by a QRS complex
    P-R interval: greater than 0.20 sec
Evaluate the patient's hemodynamic parameters: CVP, PAP,
PCWP, and CO (I)
Evaluate circulatory pressure and volume through vital signs
(I)
Measure intake, output, and specific gravity (I)
Regulate the IV flow rate (I)

Aeration
Administer humidified oxygen via mask, nasal catheter, or
nasal prongs at the prescribed flow rate (D)
Create an environment conducive to rest and sleep (I)

Nutrition
   Determine those patient's food preferences that comply
      with his or her dietary restrictions (I)
   Encourage the patient to maintain the prescribed diet (I)
   Provide a spiritual support system (I)

Communication
   Listen to the patient's concerns (I)
   Reduce the patient's anxiety level (I)
   Inform the family regarding the patient's condition (I)

Activity
   Encourage passive and active range-of-motion exercises (I)
   Encourage physical activity (I)
   Provide diversional activities (I)

Pain
   Administer analgesics to relieve any discomfort or pain (D)

Bibliography

Andreoli, K., Fowkes, V., Zipes, D., & Wallace, A. *Comprehensive cardiac care.* St. Louis: C. V. Mosby, 1979.

Shepard, N., Vaughan, P., & Rice, V. A guide to arrhythmia interpretation and management. *Critical Care Nurse,* 58-85, September-October 1982.

Zipes, D. Specific arrhythmias: Diagnosis and treatment in Braunwald, E. (ed.), *Heart disease: A textbook of cardiovascular medicine.* Philadelphia: W. B. Saunders, 1984. pp. 683-743.

Atrial-Ventricular Conduction Alteration, Mobitz Type I (Wenckeback) Second-Degree Block

DEFINITION
A Mobitz Type I (Wenckeback) second-degree A-V block produces a prolongation of the P-R interval until a sinus impulse fails to conduct through the A-V junctional tissues.

ETIOLOGY
   Inferior myocardial infarction
   Digitalis toxicity
   Myocarditis
   Occurs during sleep

A–V node degeneration
Coronary artery disease

DEFINING CHARACTERISTICS

Regulatory Behaviors
Palpitations
Dizziness
Dyspnea
Weakness
Fatigue
Syncope
A-wave in the jugular vein
S_1 faint

Cognitive Behaviors
Anxiety
Apprehension
Nervousness

NURSING RESPONSIBILITIES

Assessment
Assess regulatory behaviors indicative of Mobitz Type I
block (I)
Assess cognitive behaviors indicative of Mobitz Type I
block (I)
Monitor the ECG pattern continuously, including the pace-
maker pattern (I)
Auscultate the heart, noting any abnormal heart sounds (I)

Interventions

Fluid
Administer prescribed medications (D)
Atropine
Isoproterenol
Obtain the digitalis blood level, if applicable (D)
Interpret laboratory studies (I)
Regulate the IV flow rate (I)
Evaluate circulatory pressure and volume through vital signs
(I)
Evaluate hemodynamic parameters: PAP, PCWP, CVP, and
CO (I)

Measure the ECG components reflecting Mobitz Type I
(Wenckeback) second-degree A–V block (I)

> P–P interval: regular
>
> R–R internal: irregular
>
> P–R interval: lengths between consecutively conducted
> beats until a QRS is dropped (a P wave appears
> without a QRS complex)
>
> R–R interval: progressively shortens as the P–R inter-
> val lengthens

Inspect the jugular veins (I)

Aeration

Administer humidified oxygen via mask, nasal catheter, or
nasal prongs at the prescribed flow rate (D)

Provide an environment conducive to rest and sleep (I)

Encourage the patient to rest between nursing activities (I)

Nutrition

Encourage the patient to maintain the prescribed diet (I)

Determine those patient's food preferences that comply
with his or her dietary restrictions (I)

Provide effective oral hygiene (I)

Communication

Provide knowledge regarding diagnostic treatments and/or
supportive devices (I)

Listen to the patient's concerns regarding the causes of
arrhythmia (I)

Listen to the patient's concerns regarding possible lifestyle
changes or financial loss (I)

Reduce the patient's anxiety level (I)

Activity

Encourage passive and active range-of-motion exercises (I)

Provide follow-up care for the patient who requires a pacemaker (I)

> Inspect the surgical site for bleeding or drainage
>
> Change the dressing

Position the patient to maintain comfort and support (I)

Help the patient to increase physical activity (I)

Pain

Administer analgesics to relieve any discomfort (D)

Bibliography

Andreoli, K., Fowkes, V., Zipes, D., & Wallace, A. *Comprehensive cardiac care.* St. Louis: C. V. Mosby, 1979.

Shepard, N., Vaughan, P., & Rice, V. A guide to arrhythmia interpretation and management. *Critical Care Nurse*, 58-85, September-October 1982.

Zipes, D. Specific arrhythmias: Diagnosis and treatment in Braunwald, E. (ed.), *Heart disease: A textbook of cardiovascular medicine.* Philadelphia: W. B. Saunders, 1984, pp. 683-743.

Atrial-Ventricular Conduction Alteration, Mobitz Type II Second-Degree A-V Block

DEFINITION

A Mobitz Type II second-degree A-V block is almost always associated with a delay in conduction below the Bundle of His, in the bundle branches or in the Purkinje system.

ETIOLOGY

Rheumatic myocarditis
Coronary artery disease
A-V node degeneration
Medications
    Digitalis
    Beta blockers
    Calcium antagonist
    Quinidine
    Procainamide
    Potassium chloride
Acute myocardial infarction (anteroseptal)
Infections
    Diphtheria
    Pneumonia
    Scarlet fever
    Measles
    Mumps
    Syphilis
Bacterial endocarditis

DEFINING CHARACTERISTICS

Regulatory Behaviors
Dizziness
Fainting
Stokes-Adams attack
A waves in jugular neck vein occur intermittently, without
a subsequent carotid pulsation
Dyspnea
Weakness
Fatigue
Hypotension

Cognitive Behaviors
Confusion
Apprehension
Anxiousness

NURSING RESPONSIBILITIES

Assessment
Assess regulatory behaviors indicative of Mobitz Type 2
block (I)
Assess cognitive behaviors indicative of Mobitz Type 2
block (I)
Monitor the ECG pattern continuously for possible progres-
sion to a complete heart block (I)
Assess the side or therapeutic effects of prescribed medica-
cations (I)
Inspect the jugular veins (I)
Auscultate the heart for abnormal heart sounds (I)
Auscultate the chest for adventitious breath sounds (I)

Intervention

Fluid
Administer prescribed medications (D)
    Atropine
    Isuprel
Measure those components of the ECG reflecting a Mobitz
Type 2 block (I)
        P-P interval: regular
        R-R interval: regular or irregular

P–R interval: constant
Every P wave is not followed by a QRS complex
QRS complex: usually wide
Interpret laboratory studies (I)
Evaluate circulatory pressure and volume through vital signs (I)
Regulate the IV flow rate and maintain patency (I)
Evaluate the patient's hemodynamic parameters: PAP, PCWP, CVP, and CO (I)

Aeration

Administer humidified oxygen via mask, nasal catheter, or nasal prongs at the prescribed flow rate (I)
Provide an environment conducive to rest and sleep (I)
Encourage the patient to rest between nursing activities (I)

Nutrition

Encourage the patient to maintain the prescribed low-salt diet (I)
Determine those patient's food preferences that comply with his or her dietary restrictions (I)
Provide a spiritual support system (I)

Communication

Provide knowledge regarding diagnostic studies (I)
Provide knowledge regarding the probable prophylactic use of a pacemaker (I)
Listen to the patient's concerns (I)
Reduce the patient's anxiety level (I)

Activity

Encourage passive and active range-of-motion exercises (I)
Provide postoperative follow-up care for the patient requiring a pacemaker (I)
Inspect the surgical site for bleeding or drainage (I)
Change dressings q4h or as necessary to prevent infection (I)
Position the patient to maintain comfort and support (I)
Help the patient to gradually increase his or her physical activity (I)

Pain

Determine the type, location, and duration of pain (I)
Administer analgesics to relieve discomfort (I)

Bibliography

Andreoli, K., Fowkes, V., Zipes, D., & Wallace, A. *Comprehensive cardiac care.* St. Louis: C. V. Mosby, 1979.

Shepard, N., Vaughan, P., & Rice, V. A guide to arrhythmia interpretation and management. *Critical Care Nurse,* 58-85, September-October 1982.

Zipes, D. Specific arrhythmias: Diagnosis and treatment in Braunwald, E. (ed.), *Heart disease: A textbook of cardiovascular medicine.* Philadelphia: W. B. Saunders, 1984, pp. 683-743.

Atrial-Ventricular Conduction Alteration, Complete Heart Block

DEFINITION

Complete A-V block results when all of the supraventricular impulses are blocked or interrupted within the conduction system, thus failing to reach and activate the ventricular myocardium.

ETIOLOGY

Acute myocardial infarction
> Inferior wall MI
>> A complete A-V block is intranodal, with a 25-percent mortality rate
> Anterior MI
>> A complete A-V block is a manifestation of a bilateral bundle branch block, with a high mortality rate

Aortic stenosis
Degeneration of the conduction system
> Lev's disease
> Lenegre's disease

Cardiac surgery

DEFINING CHARACTERISTICS

Regulatory Behaviors

Weakness
Faintness
Dyspnea
Angina
Syncope

Slow ventricular rate < 50 bpm

A waves in jugular veins occur independently of V waves or carotid pulsations

Cannon a-waves occur with simultaneous atrial and ventricular contractions S_1

Unusually loud when atrial contraction immediately precedes ventricular contraction

Faint when atrial contraction precedes ventricular contraction by a long period of time

Cognitive Behaviors

Anxiety

Apprehension

Restlessness

Confusion

Loss of consciousness

NURSING RESPONSIBILITIES

Assessment

Assess regulatory behaviors reflective of a complete A–V block (I)

Assess cognitive behaviors reflective of a complete A–V block (I)

Monitor the ECG pattern continuously, including the pacemaker pattern (I)

Observe the side or therapeutic effects of prescribed medications (I)

Inspect the jugular veins (I)

Auscultate the heart for abnormal heart sounds (I)

Auscultate the chest for adventitious breath sounds (I)

Interventions

Fluid

Administer prescribed medications (D)

Atropine

Isuprel

Epinephrine

Measure the ECG components reflecting a complete A–V block (I)

P–P interval: regular

R–R interval: regular
P–R interval: varies
Atrial rate: greater than the ventricular rate
Evaluate laboratory studies (I)
Evaluate circulatory pressure and volume through vital signs (I)
Regulate the IV flow rate and maintain patency (I)
Evaluate the patient's hemodynamic parameters: PAP, PCWP, CVP, and CO (I)

Aeration
Administer humidified oxygen via mask, nasal catheter, or nasal prongs at the prescribed flow rate (I)
Provide an environment conducive to rest and sleep (I)
Encourage the patient to rest between nursing activities (I)

Nutrition
Encourage the patient to maintain the prescribed low-salt diet (I)
Determine those patients's food preferences that comply with his or her dietary restrictions (I)
Provide a spiritual support system (I)

Communication
Provide knowledge regarding diagnostic studies (I)
Provide knowledge regarding the probable prophylactic use of a pacemaker (I)
Listen to the patient's concerns (I)
Reduce the patient's anxiety level (I)

Activity
Encourage passive and active range-of-motion exercises (I)
Provide postoperative follow-up care for the patient requiring a pacemaker (I)
Inspect the surgical site for bleeding or drainage (I)
Change dressings q4h or as necessary to prevent infection (I)
Position the patient to maintain comfort and support (I)
Assist the patient to gradually increase physical activity (I)
Provide postoperative follow-up care for the patient requiring an epicardial or a permanent transvenous pacemaker (I)

Pain
Administer the prescribed analgesics (D)
Determine the type, location, and duration of pain (I)

Bibliography

Andreoli, K., Fowkes, V., Zipes, D., & Wallace, A. *Comprehensive cardiac care.* St. Louis: C. V. Mosby, 1979.

Shepard, N., Vaughan, P., & Rice, V. A guide to arrhythmia interpretation and management. *Critical Care Nurse,* 58–85, September–October 1982.

Zipes, D. Specific arrhythmias: Diagnosis and treatment in Braunwald, E. (ed.), *Heart disease: A textbook of cardiovascular medicine.* Philadelphia: W. B. Saunders, 1984, 683–743.

Ventricular Conduction Alteration, Premature Ventricular Beat

DEFINITION

A premature ventricular beat (PVB) is characterized by the premature occurrence of the QRS complex arising below the bifurcation of the bundle of His, from the bundle branches or from the Purkinje network.

ETIOLOGY

Fatigue
Emotional distress
Caffeine
Tobacco
Drug toxicity
Hypokalemia
Hypoxia
Myocardial ischemia
Manipulation of heart tissue
Myocardial infarction

DEFINING CHARACTERISTICS

Regulatory Behaviors
Sensation of skipped beats
Palpitations
Discomfort in the chest or the neck

Angina

Hypokalemia

Decreased cardiac output

Decreased stroke volume, resulting in a faintly palpable
radial pulse (I)

Cannon A waves in the jugular veins (I)

Cognitive Behaviors

Anxiousness

Apprehension

Nervousness

NURSING RESPONSIBILITIES

Assessment

Assess regulatory behaviors indicative of PVB (I)

Assess cognitive behaviors indicative of PVB (I)

Monitor the ECG pattern continuously (I)

Observe the side or therapeutic effects of prescribed medications (I)

Assess the types of PVB: unifocal, multifocal, and variable
coupling (I)

Auscultate the heart for abnormal heart sounds (I)

Inspect the jugular veins (I)

Auscultate the chest for adventitious breath sounds (I)

Interventions

Fluid

Administer prescribed medications (D)

IV bolus of lidocaine:

50–100 mg IV

IV drip 1–4 mg/min

Pronestyl

Quinidine

Propranolol

Bretylol

Measure the ECG components reflecting PVB (I)

QRS complex: early, wide, bizarre

No associated P wave

Compensatory pause: usually complete

Evaluate laboratory studies (I)

Evaluate circulatory pressure and volume through vital signs (I)

Regulate the IV flow rate and maintain patency (I)

Evaluate the patient's hemodynamic parameters: PAP, PCWP, CVP, and CO (I)

Aeration

Administer humidified oxygen via mask, nasal catheter, or nasal prongs at the prescribed flow rate (D)

Provide an environment conducive to rest and sleep (I)

Encourage the patient to rest between nursing activities (I)

Nutrition

Encourage the patient to maintain the prescribed low-salt diet (I)

Provide a spiritual support system (I)

Communication

Provide knowledge regarding diagnostic studies (I)

Listen to the patient's concerns (I)

Reduce the patient's anxiety level (I)

Activity

Encourage passive and active range-of-motion exercises (I)

Position the patient to maintain comfort and support (I)

Pain

Administer analgesics to relieve discomfort (D)

Determine the type, location, and duration of pain (I)

Bibliography

Andreoli, K., Fowkes, V., Zipes, D., & Wallace, A. *Comprehensive cardiac care.* St. Louis: C. V. Mosby, 1979.

Shepard, N., Vaughan, P., & Rice, V. A guide to arrhythmia interpretation and management. *Critical Care Nurse,* 58–85, September–October 1982.

Zipes, D. Specific arrhythmias: Diagnosis and treatment in Braunwald, E. (ed.), *Heart disease: A textbook of cardiovascular medicine.* Philadelphia: W. B. Saunders, 1984, 683–743.

Ventricular Conduction Alteration, Ventricular Tachycardia

DEFINITION
Ventricular tachycardia (VT) is defined as the consecutive appearance of three or more ectopic ventricular beats at a rate greater than 100 bpm, with a QRS morphology similar to that of ventricular premature beats.

ETIOLOGY
Myocardial infarction
Ischemic heart disease
    Angina
    Congestive heart failure
    Left ventricular aneurysm
Coronary artery disease
Mitral valve prolapse
Brady-tachy syndrome
Cardiomyopathy
Valve disease
Myocarditis
Drug toxicity

DEFINING CHARACTERISTICS

Regulatory Behaviors
Weakness
Dizziness
Syncope
Angina
Shortness of breath
Hypotension
Rapid, thready, and regular radial pulse
S_4
S_3
Cannon A waves in the jugular veins

Cognitive Behaviors
Anxiousness
Apprehension
Nervousness
Restlessness

NURSING RESPONSIBILITIES

Assessment

Assess regulatory behaviors indicative of VT (I)

Assess cognitive behaviors indicative of VT (I)

Monitor the ECG pattern continuously (I)

Assess the side or therapeutic effects of prescribed medications (I)

Auscultate the heart for abnormal heart sounds (I)

Inspect the jugular veins (I)

Auscultate the chest for adventitious breath sounds (I)

Auscultate the chest for rate, rhythm, and regularity (I)

Interventions

Fluid

Administer prescribed medications (D)

    Lidocaine

        75–100 mg IV (repeated q3–5 min)

        2–4 mg/min

    Procainamide

    Propranolol

    Quinidine

    Diphenylhydantoin

    Disopyramide

    Bretylium tosylate

Measure the ECG components reflective of VT (I)

    QRS complexes: wide and bizarre

    No associated P waves

    R–R interval: usually regular

    Ventricular rate: over 100 bpm

Evaluate laboratory studies (I)

Evaluate circulatory pressure and volume through vital signs (I)

Regulate the IV flow rate and maintain patency (I)

Aeration

Provide an environment conducive to rest and sleep (I)

Nutrition

Encourage the patient to maintain the prescribed low-salt diet (I)

Provide a spiritual support system (I)

Communication
   Provide knowledge regarding diagnostic studies (I)
   Assist the physician as he or she explains the purposes of
      intracardiac pacing (I)
   Listen to the patient's concerns (I)
   Reduce the patient's anxiety level (I)

Activity
   Assist the physician with cardioversion (D)
   Encourage passive and active range-of-motion exercises (I)
   Position the patient to maintain comfort and support (I)

Pain
   Determine the type, location, and duration of pain (I)
   Administer analgesics to relieve any discomfort (I)

Bibliography

Andreoli, K., Fowkes, V., Zipes, D., & Wallace, A. *Comprehensive
   cardiac care*. St. Louis: C. V. Mosby, 1979.
Shepard, N., Vaughan, P., & Rice, V. A guide to arrhythmia interpre-
   tation and management. *Critical Care Nurse*, 58–85, September–
   October 1982.
Zipes, D. Specific arrhythmias: Diagnosis and treatment in Braunwald,
   E. (ed.), *Heart disease: A textbook of cardiovascular medicine*.
   Philadelphia: W. B. Saunders, 1984, 683–743.

Ventricular Conduction Alteration, Ventricular Fibrillation

DEFINITION
Ventricular fibrillation represents uncoordinated, chaotic
depolarization of the ventricles.

ETIOLOGY
   Coronary artery disease
   Coronary spasm
   Myocardial disease
   Valve disease
   Drug toxicity
   Electrolyte disturbance

DEFINING CHARACTERISTICS

Regulatory Behaviors
Palpitations
Chest pain
Absence of pulses
No palpitable blood pressure
Cyanosis
Dilated pupils
Convulsions
Incontinence
Apnea

Cognitive Behaviors
Restlessness
Apprehension
Anxiousness
Confusion
Altered mental state

NURSING RESPONSIBILITIES

Assessment
Assess regulatory behaviors indicative of ventricular fibrillation (I)
Assess cognitive behaviors indicative of ventricular fibrillation (I)
Monitor the ECG pattern continuously (I)
Assess the side or therapeutic effects of prescribed medications (I)
Auscultate the heart for abnormal heart sounds (I)
Inspect the skin for cyanosis (I)

Interventions

Fluid
Administer prescribed medications (D)
Adrenalin
Bretylol
Lidocaine
Administer the prescribed IV fluids (D)

Measure the ECG components reflective of ventricular
fibrillation (I)
   Baseline: wavy, undulating
   P Waves: absent
   QRS complex: absent
Evaluate laboratory studies for metabolic acidosis (I)
Check for the presence/absence of peripheral pulses and for
bilateral equality (I)
Evaluate circulatory pressure and volume through vital
signs (I)
Measure intake and output (I)

Aeration

Maintain a patent airway (I)
Provide ventilatory support to maintain respiratory stabil-
ity (I)
Evaluate arterial blood gasses for respiratory acidosis and/or
hypoxemia (I)
Evaluate the effectiveness of ventilatory support (I)

Nutrition

Withhold food and drink until ventricular fibrillation has
stabilized (I)

Communication

Inform the family of any changes in the patient's cardiac
status (I)
Reduce both patient and family anxiety levels (I)
Provide knowledge regarding the sudden need for supportive
devices (I)

Activity

Initiate cardiac resuscitation (I)
Assist the physician with defibrillation (ID)
Immobilize the patient until the origin of ventricular fibril-
lation can be determined (I)

Pain

Administer analgesics, when realistic (D)
Determine whether or not the patient experienced pain
prior to the ventricular fibrillation episode (I)

Bibliography

Andreoli, K., Fowkes, V., Zipes, D., & Wallace, A. *Comprehensive cardiac care*. St. Louis: C. V. Mosby, 1979.

Shepard, N., Vaughan, P., & Rice, V. A guide to arrhythmia interpretation and management. *Critical Care Nurse*, 58–85, September–October 1982.

Zipes, D. Specific arrhythmias: Diagnosis and treatment in Braunwald, E. (ed.), *Heart disease: A textbook of cardiovascular medicine*. Philadelphia: W. B. Saunders, 1984, 683–743.

Ventricular Conduction Alteration, Accelerated Idioventricular Rhythm

DEFINITION

The ventricular rate, commonly between 50 and 110 bpm, usually hovers within 10 beats of the sinus rate; control of the cardiac rhythm may be passed back and forth between these two competing pacemaker sites.

ETIOLOGY

Acute myocardial infarction

Digitalis toxicity

DEFINING CHARACTERISTICS

Regulatory Behaviors

Decreased cardiac output
    Dizziness
    Hypotension
    Weak peripheral pulses
    Dyspnea
Decreased stroke volume

Cognitive Behaviors

Anxiousness
Nervousness
Apprehension

NURSING RESPONSIBILITIES

Assessment

Assess regulatory behaviors indicative of accelerated idioventricular arrhythmia (I)

Assess cognitive behaviors indicative of accelerated idioventricular arrhythmia (I)

Monitor the ECG pattern continuously (I)

Observe the side or therapeutic effects of prescribed medications (I)

Inspect the jugular veins (I)

Auscultate the heart for abnormal heart sounds (I)

Auscultate the chest for adventitious breath sounds (I)

Interventions

Fluid

Administer prescribed medications (D)

Type 2 accelerated ventricular rhythm
Lidocaine
Pronestyl
Norpace
Inderal
Quinidine
Bretylium

Administer the prescribed IV fluids (D)

Measure the ECG components reflective of ventricular fibrillation (I)
QRS complexes: wide and bizarre
No associated P waves
R–R interval: regular
Ventricular rate: 40–100 bpm

Regulate the IV flow rate and check patency (I)

Differentiate Type 1 accelerated ventricular rhythm (benign escape rhythm initiated by a ventricular escape beat) from Type 2 accelerated ventricular rhythm (irritable ventricular ectopic rhythm, which can progress to ventricular tachycardia) (I)

Evaluate laboratory studies (I)

Measure arterial blood pressure (I)

Evaluate hemodynamic parameters, if available: PAP, PCWP, CVP, and CO (I)

Measure intake and output (I)

Aeration

Administer humidified oxygen via mask, nasal catheter, or nasal prongs at the prescribed flow rate (I)

Provide an environment conducive to rest and sleep (I)

Nutrition

Withhold food and drink until arrhythmia stabilizes (I)

Provide a spiritual support system (I)

Comminication

Provide knowledge regarding diagnostic studies (I)

Listen to the patient's concerns (I)

Reduce the patient's anxiety level (I)

Activity

Encourage passive and active range-of-motion exercises (I)

Pain

Administer analgesics to relieve pain (D)

Determine the type, location, and duration of pain (I)

Bibliography

Andreoli, K., Fowkes, V., Zipes, D., & Wallace, A. *Comprehensive cardiac care*. St. Louis: C. V. Mosby, 1979.

Shepard, N., Vaughan, P., & Rice, V. A guide to arrhythmia interpretation and management. *Critical Care Nurse*, 58–85, September–October 1982.

Zipes, D. Specific arrhythmias: Diagnosis and treatment in Braunwald, E. (ed.), *Heart disease: A textbook of cardiovascular medicine*. Philadelphia: W. B. Saunders, 1984, 683–743.

FLUID-VOLUME DEFICIT

Actual Whole Blood-Volume Deficit, Hemorrhagic Shock

DEFINITION

Loss of 30–50 percent of whole blood volume in a previously healthy person in circulatory failure and manifestations of profound shock.

ETIOLOGY
Arterial injury
Venous injury
Fractures
Open
Femur
Tibia
Closed
Pelvis
Spine
Femur shaft

DEFINING CHARACTERISTICS

Regulatory Behaviors
Tachycardia
Tachypnea
Thirst
Pallor
Cool, dry skin
Oliguria
Bluish nail beds
Rales
Weakness
Increased PAP
Increased PCWP
Dizziness
Cyanosis

Cognitive Behaviors
Apprehension
Restlessness
Confusion
Dulled sensorium
Listlessness
Stupor
Unconsciousness

NURSING RESPONSIBILITIES

Assessment
Assess regulatory behaviors indicative of hemorrhagic
shock (I)

Assess cognitive behaviors indicative of hemorrhagic shock (I)

Monitor the ECG pattern continuously (I)

Assess the patient's neurological status (I)

Observe the side or therapeutic effects of prescribed medications (I)

Inspect the skin for bruising, petechiae, or other hemorrhagic signs (I)

Inspect the color of the stools (I)

Inspect the source of overt bleeding (I)

Auscultate the heart for rate, rhythm, and regularity (I)

Auscultate the heart for abnormal heart sounds (I)

Auscultate the chest for abnormal breath sounds (I)

Inspect the skin for pallor or cyanosis (I)

Interventions

Fluid

Administer the prescribed IV fluids (D)
> Whole blood
> Ringer's lactate
> Albumin

Evaluate the skin for color, turgor, and temperature (I)

Evaluate capillary refill time (I)

Evaluate orthostatic vital signs, including blood pressure and pulse (I)

Evaluate data from hemodynamic parameters: CVP, PAP, PCWP, SVR, and CO (I)

Measure urinary volume and specific gravity (I)

Measure the amount of drainage from tubes (I)

Evaluate hematocrit, hemoglobin, white blood cell (WBC) differentials, and coagulation panel (I)

Measure intake (I)

Aeration

Provide oxygen via mask, nasal catheter, or nasal prongs at the prescribed percentage or flow rate (D)

Evaluate the breathing pattern for shortness of breath or dyspnea (I)

Reduce meaningless or stressful environmental stimuli during the initial crisis (I)

Suction the patient via mouth or endotracheal tube while using strict aseptic techniques (I)

Evaluate the presence of blood in the tracheal aspirate (I)
Evaluate chest movement for symmetry (I)

Nutrition
Nothing by mouth (NPO)

Communication
Instruct both patient and family in the signs and symptoms
   of impending shock (I)
Instruct the patient in signs and symptoms of the specific
   type of bleeding problem affecting him or her (I)
Reduce the patient's anxiety level (I)
Inform the physician of any changes in the patient's condi-
   tion (I)

Activity
Measure abdominal girth (I)
Position the patient so that there is adequate blood flow to
   the brain: supine position, with legs elevated on pillows
   at a 20 to 30-degree angle (I)
Evaluate any alterations in the thought process (I)
Place the patient on complete bed rest until his or her vital
   signs stabilize (I)
Position the patient so that he or she is comfortable (I)

Pain
Administer prescribed analgesics (D)
Evaluate for abdominal discomfort (I)

Bibliography
Bordicks, K. *Pattern of shock implications for nursing care.* New York:
   Macmillan, 1980.
Gettrust, K., Ryan, S., & Engleman, D. *Applied nursing diagnosis.* New
   York: Wiley, 1985.

RESPIRATORY SYSTEM

The critical care nurse derives several collaborative nursing
diagnoses by assessing the patient's respiratory status. The
nurse inspects for signs of respiratory distress; palpates the
chest for a possible abnormality in excursion, symmetry, or

fremitus; auscultates the chest for adventitious breath sounds; and percusses the chest.

FLUID-VOLUME EXCESS
Extracellular Fluid-Volume Excess, Alveolar Edema

DEFINITION
Alveolar edema is an excessive volume of blood in the pulmonary venous bed, the term implies that fluid is moved from the capillaries into the interstitial spaces of the lungs and alveoli.

ETIOLOGY
  Cardiogenic
    Left ventricular failure
    Myocardial infarction
    Mitral stenosis and insufficiency
    Arterial hypertension
    Volume overload
  Altered permeability of pulmonary capillary membrane
    Inhaled toxic elements
    Adult respiratory distress syndrome
    Bacteremic sepsis
    Uremia
    Disseminated intravascular coagulation
    Mechanical ventilation
    Aspiration
  Decreased plasma oncotic pressure, hypoproteinemia
    Starvation
    Hepatic cirrhosis
    Nephrotic syndrome
    Hemorrhage
    Lymphatic obstruction
  Other
    High-altitude pulmonary edema
    Heroin overdose
    Neurogenic edema
    Pulmonary embolism
    Postanesthetic edema

DEFINING CHARACTERISTICS

Regulatory Behaviors
Persistent cough
Dyspnea
Orthopnea
Exercise intolerance
Crepitant rales
Diastolic gallop
Shortness of breath
Frothy, blood-tinged sputum
Cyanosis
Diaphoresis
Tachycardia
Hypotension

Cognitive Behaviors
Confusion
Restlessness
Anxiousness
Altered memory
Noncompliance
Lethargy

NURSING RESPONSIBILITIES

Assessment
Assess regulatory behaviors indicative of alveolar edema (I)
Assess cognitive behaviors indicative of alveolar edema (I)
Monitor the ECG pattern continuously (I)
Observe the side or therapeutic effects of prescribed medications (I)
Auscultate the heart for abnormal heart sounds (I)
Palpate for the presence of peripheral pulses and check for bilateral equality (I)
Inspect the extremities for edema (I)
Auscultate the chest for adventitious breath sounds (I)
Palpate the chest for tactile fremitus (I)
Inspect the skin color for pallor, dusky-ashen features, or cyanosis (I)
Inspect chest movement for labored breathing and symmetry (I)

Auscultate the chest for respiratory rate, rhythm, and regularity (I)

Interventions

Fluids

Administer IV albumin at the prescribed flow rate (D)
Administer prescribed medications (D)
    Morphine sulfate
    Lasix
    Edecrin
    Aminophylline
    Digitalis
    Deslanoside (Cedilanid D)
    Ovabain (G-Strophanthin)
    Nitroglycerin
    Nitroprusside
    Phentolamine
Regulate the IV flow rate and check for patency (I)
Evaluate the data from hemodynamic parameters: PAP, PCWP, CVP, and CO (I)
Measure arterial blood pressure and MAP (I)
Measure intake, output, specific gravity, and daily weight (I)
Compare apical and radial pulses (I)
Evaluate the patient's skin for temperature changes and diaphoresis (I)
Evaluate the results of pulmonary function tests (vital capacity, functional residual volume, total lung capacity, tidal volume, minute volume, forced vital capacity, and compliance (I)
Evaluate arterial blood gasses (I)
Evaluate the jugular veins for distention (I)

Aeration

Review with the physician the patient's chest film (ID)
Provide humidified oxygen via mask, nasal catheter, or nasal prongs at the prescribed flow rate (I)
Encourage the patient to deep-breathe and cough (I)
Provide ventilatory support as needed (I)

Evaluate the patient's compatibility with ventilatory support: mode, frequency, PEEP, and synchrony (I)

Remove mucous and secretions from the respiratory tract (I)

Nutrition

Restrict fluid intake (ID)

Encourage the patient to maintain the prescribed low-salt diet (I)

Assist the patient with eating (I)

Provide a spiritual support system (I)

Create an environment conducive to eating (I)

Communication

Listen to the patient's concerns and fears (I)

Provide knowledge regarding diagnostic procedures and supportive devices (I)

Inform the physician of any significant changes in the patient's condition and of the results of laboratory studies (I)

Provide knowledge regarding illness and prognosis (I)

Relieve distress related to invasive procedures (I)

Support the family through the patient's hospitalization (I)

Activity

Apply rotating tourniquets as needed (ID)

    Check for the presence of peripheral pulses, and check temperature and color of the extremities

    Rotate cuffs in sequence q15 min

    Observe for edema, pain, and/or loss of function in any extremity

    Remove the tourniquets by rotating off one at a time at 15-min intervals

Reduce the patient's anxiety level (I)

Increase positional tolerance by gradually turning and/or positioning the patient in order to provide adequate ventilation (I)

Place the patient in the high Fowler's position, with lower legs dependent (I)

Provide support for increasing physical activity (I)

Evaluate any alterations in the thought process (I)

Pain
  Administer analgesics as prescribed (D)
  Evaluate the type, location, and duration of pain (I)

Bibliography
Borg, N., Nikas, D., Stark, J., & Williams, S. *Core curriculum critical care nursing*. Philadelphia: W. B. Saunders, 1981.
Johanson, B., Dungca, C., Hoffmeister, D., & Wells, S. *Standards for critical care* (2nd ed.). St. Louis: C. V. Mosby, 1985.
Roberts, S. *Physiological concepts and the critically ill patient*. Englewood Cliffs, N.J.: Prentice-Hall, 1985, pp. 134–176.

ACID-BASE IMBALANCE

Carbon Dioxide Gas Exchange, Impaired, Respiratory Acidosis

DEFINITION
Respiratory acidosis is an elevated arterial PCO_2 that causes an increase in hydrogen ion and thus a decrease in pH.

ETIOLOGY
  Alveolar hypoventilation
    Pulmonary disease
    Overdose of drugs
    Obesity
    Mechanical asphyxia
    Sleep
    CNS lesion
    Impaired respiratory muscles

DEFINING CHARACTERISTICS

Regulatory Behaviors
  Tachycardia
  Dyspnea
  Tachypnea
  Diaphoresis
  Cyanosis
  Arrhythmias

Cognitive Behaviors
  Restlessness
  Confusion
  Lethargy
  Coma

NURSING RESPONSIBILITIES

Assessment

  Assess regulatory behaviors indicative of respiratory acidosis (I)
  Assess cognitive behaviors indicative of respiratory acidosis (I)
  Monitor the ECG pattern continuously (I)
  Assess the patient's neurological status (I)
  Auscultate the heart for abnormal heart sounds (I)
  Auscultate the chest for adventitious breath sounds (I)
  Inspect for dyspnea (I)
  Auscultate the chest for respiratory rate, rhythm, and regularity (I)

Interventions

Fluid

  Administer prescribed medications (D)
    Bicarbonate
    Diuretics
  Administer prescribed IV fluids (D)
  Measure arterial blood pressure and MAP (I)
    Evaluate the skin for color, temperature, and diaphoresis (I)
  Measure intake, output, and specific gravity (I)
  Evaluate laboratory studies (I)

Aeration

  Provide humidified oxygen at the prescribed flow rate (D)
  Evaluate the skin for cyanosis (I)
  Provide ventilatory support as needed (I)
  Establish and maintain a patent airway (I)
  Evaluate for airway obstruction (I)
  Remove mucous and secretions from respiratory tract (I)

Nutrition
Withhold food until the patient is able to eat (I)
Consult with both physician and dietitian (I)

Communication
Listen to the patient's concerns, fears, and anxieties (I)
Reduce the patient's anxiety level (I)
Encourage self-performance, when possible (I)
Inform the physician of changes in the patient's condition
and of the results of laboratory studies (I)

Activity
Change the patient's position q2h (I)
Evaluate the patient for abnormal body movement (I)
Evaluate any alteration in the patient's thought process (I)

Pain
Administer analgesics as prescribed (D)
Estimate the degree of pain expressed (I)

Bibliography

Borg, N., Nikas, D., Stark, J., & Williams, S. *Core curriculum for critical care nursing.* Philadelphia: W. B. Saunders, 1981.

Emanuelson, K. & Densmore, M. *Acute respiratory care.* Bethany, Conn. Fleschner Publishing Company, 1981.

Wade, J. *Comprehensive respiratory care.* St. Louis: C. V. Mosby, 1982.

Carbon Dioxide Gas Exchange, Impaired, Respiratory Alkalosis

DEFINITION
Respiratory alkalosis is reduced arterial CO_2, which results in fewer hydrogen ions and bicarbonate ions and an increased pH.

ETIOLOGY
Alveolar hyperventilation
Overventilation by a ventilator
Therapeutic response to metabolic acidosis
Bacteremia
Thyrotoxicosis
Fever
Hepatic encephalopathy

Response to hypoxia
Hysteria
Ammonia intoxication
Anxiety
Salicylate intoxication
Hypoxemia
Pulmonary disease
Intrathoracic processes
Pulmonary emboli
Pneumonia
Asthma
Pulmonary fibrosis
CNS disorders
Cerebrovascular accident (CVA)
Tumor
Infection

DEFINING CHARACTERISTICS

Regulatory Behaviors
Numbness
Tingling
Muscle twitching
Tetany

Cognitive Behaviors
Nervousness
Irritability
Anxiety

NURSING RESPONSIBILITIES

Assessment
Assess regulatory behaviors indicative of respiratory alkalosis (I)
Assess cognitive behaviors indicative of respiratory alkalosis (I)
Monitor the ECG pattern continuously (I)
Auscultate the heart for abnormal heart sounds (I)
Palpate for arterial pulsations/peripheral pulses (I)
Auscultate the chest for adventitious breath sounds (I)
Inspect for shortness of breath or dyspnea (I)

Auscultate the chest for respiratory rate, rhythm, and regularity (I)

Interventions

Fluid

Administer prescribed medications (D)
Administer prescribed IV fluids (D)
Evaluate serum electrolytes (I)
Measure arterial blood pressure and MAP (I)
Measure intake, urinary volume, and specific gravity (I)

Aeration

Evaluate the setting on ventilatory support for a possible need to change the volume setting, flow rate, or delivery (ID)
Encourage the patient to breathe exhaled air from a paper bag (I)
Provide oxygen at the prescribed flow rate (I)
Provide ventilatory support as needed (I)
Evaluate the need to increase the tubing between patient and ventilator (I)
Evaluate arterial blood gasses in relationship to ventilatory therapy (I)

Nutrition

Encourage the patient to maintain the prescribed diet (I)
Consult with both physician and dietitian (I)
Assist the patient with eating (I)

Communication

Listen to the patient's concerns, fears, and anxieties (I)
Reduce the patient's anxiety level (I)
Inform the physician of any changes in the patient's condition and of the results of laboratory studies (I)
Support the family throughout the patient's hospitalization (I)
Inform the patient of arterial blood gasses indicating respiratory alkalosis (I)
Consult with both physician and respiratory therapist regarding a possible need to change the volume of ventilatory support (I)

Activity
   Change the patient's position q2h (I)
   Evaluate any alteration in the patient's thought process (I)
   Encourage alternative rest and moderate activity periods (I)

Pain
   Administer prescribed analgesics (D)
   Evaluate the degree of pain expressed (I)

Bibliography
Harper, R. *A guide to respiratory care*. Philadelphia: Lippincott, 1981.
Wade, J. *Comprehensive respiratory care*. St. Louis: C. V. Mosby, 1982.

IMPAIRED GAS EXCHANGE

Oxygen Gas Exchange, Impaired, Hypoxemia

DEFINITION
Arterial hypoxemia is deficient oxygenation of the arterial blood.

ETIOLOGY
   Altitude-low inspired PaO_2
   Alveolar hypoventilation
   Ventilation–perfusion mismatching
      Pulmonary emboli
      Shock
      Atelectasis
      Right to left shunt
      Adult respiratory distress syndrome
   Diffusion defects
      Pulmonary fibrosis
   Anatomic venous-to-arterial shunt
      Pneumonia
      Vascular lung tumor
      Intracardiac right-to-left shunt

DEFINING CHARACTERISTICS

Regulatory Behaviors
   Headache
   Tachycardia

    Cyanosis
    Tachypnea
    Arrhythmias
    Polycythemia
    Hypertension/hypotension

Cognitive Behaviors
    Change in personality
    Loss of judgment
    Inability to concentrate
    Restlessness
    Paranoia
    Anxiety

NURSING RESPONSIBILITIES

Assessment
Assess regulatory behaviors indicative of hypoxemia (I)
Assess cognitive behaviors indicative of hypoxemia (I)
Monitor the ECG pattern continuously (I)
Observe the side or therapeutic effects of prescribed medications (I)
Assess chest excursion (I)
Auscultate the heart for abnormal heart sounds (I)
Palpate for the presence of peripheral pulses and check for bilateral equality (I)
Inspect the skin for color, temperature, and presence of diaphoresis (I)
Auscultate the chest for adventitious breath sounds (I)
Inspect the skin color for pallor, dusky-ashen features, or cyanosis (I)
Auscultate the chest for respiratory rate, rhythm, and regularity (I)

Interventions

Fluid
Administer prescribed medications (D)
Instruct the patient in the use of inhaled medications (I)
Administer prescribed IV fluids (I)
Regulate the IV flow rate and check for patency (I)

Evaluate data from hemodynamic parameters: PAP, PCWP, CVP, and CO (I)

Measure arterial blood pressure and MAP (I)

Measure intake, output, specific gravity, and daily weight (I)

Aeration

Provide humidified oxygen via mask, nasal catheter, or nasal prongs at the prescribed flow rate (D)

Provide ventilatory support as needed (I)

Evaluate the patient's compatibility with ventilatory support: mode, frequency, PEEP, and synchrony (I)

Remove mucous and secretions from the respiratory tract (I)

Nutrition

Encourage the patient to maintain the prescribed diet (I)

Assist the patient with eating, if necessary (I)

Create an atmosphere conducive to eating (I)

Communication

Provide knowledge regarding illness and prognosis (ID)

Listen to the patient's concerns and fears (I)

Provide knowledge regarding diagnostic procedures and supportive devices (I)

Reduce the patient's anxiety level (I)

Support the patient throughout his or her hospitalization (I)

Activity

Provide for moderate physical activity (I)

Increase positional tolerance by gradually turning and/or positioning the patient in order to provide adequate ventilation (I)

Evaluate for altered thought process (I)

Pain

Administer analgesics as prescribed (D)

Evaluate the type, location, and duration of pain (I)

Bibliography

Carpenito, L. J. *Handbook of nursing diagnosis*. Philadelphia: Lippincott, 1984.

Gettrust, K., Ryan, S., & Engleman, D. *Applied nursing diagnosis*. New York: Wiley, 1985.

Kelly, M. *Nursing diagnosis source book*. Norwalk, Conn.: Appleton-Century-Crofts, 1985.

Kim, M. J., McFarland, G., & McLane, A. *Nursing diagnosis*. St. Louis: C. V. Mosby, 1984.

Carbon Dioxide Gas Exchange, Impaired, Hypercapnia

DEFINITION

Hypercapnia is defined as carbon dioxide retention and elevation of PCO_2 in alveoli and arterial blood.

ETIOLOGY

Decreased respiratory drive
    Drug intoxication
    Cerebral trauma
Neuromuscular disorders
    Spinal injury
    Myasthenia gravis
    Multiple sclerosis
Adult respiratory distress syndrome
    Shock
    Fat emboli
    Pulmonary emboli
Airway obstruction
    Chronic bronchitis
    Emphysema
    Asthma
    Tumor
Impaired diaphragmatic movement
    Trauma
    Paralysis
Impaired diffusion
    Pulmonary fibrosis
    Destruction of pulmonary capillary bed

DEFINING CHARACTERISTICS

Regulatory Behaviors
Hypotension
Tachycardia

Hyperventilation
Warm, diaphoretic skin
Headache
Drowsiness
Asterixis
Cyanosis
Lethargy
Coma

Cognitive Behaviors

Inability to concentrate
Lack of judgment
Irritability
Altered sleep pattern
Hallucination

NURSING RESPONSIBILITIES

Assessment

Assess regulatory behaviors indicative of hypercapnia (I)
Assess cognitive behaviors indicative of hypercapnia (I)
Monitor the ECG pattern continuously (I)
Assess the patient's neurological status (I)
Observe the side or therapeutic effects of prescribed medications (I)
Auscultate the heart for abnormal heart sounds (I)
Palpate for arterial pulsations/peripheral pulses (I)
Inspect extremities for edema (I)
Inspect the jugular veins (I)
Palpate the point of maximum cardiac impulse, or point of maximum intensity (PMI) (I)
Auscultate the chest for adventitious breath sounds (I)
Inspect for dyspnea (I)
Palpate the chest for tactile fremitus (I)
Auscultate the chest for respiratory rate, rhythm, and regularity (I)
Percuss the chest for abnormal resonance (I)
Auscultate the chest for normal breath sounds: bronchial, vesicular, and bronchovesicular (I)

Interventions

Fluid

Administer prescribed medications (D)

Evaluate data from hemodynamic parameters: PAP, PCWP, CVP, and CO (I)

Measure arterial blood pressure and MAP (I)

Evaluate the patient's skin for temperature change and diaphoresis (I)

Measure intake, output, and specific gravity (I)

Evaluate urine for abnormal color, content, and odor (I)

Evaluate laboratory studies (I)

Aeration

Provide oxygen at the prescribed flow rate (D)

Evaluate the skin for cyanosis (I)

Encourage the patient to cough, turn, and deep-breathe (I)

Provide ventilatory support as needed (I)

Establish and maintain a patent airway (I)

Evaluate for airway obstruction (I)

Remove mucous and secretions from the respiratory tract (I)

Nutrition

Withhold food until after the patient has been able to rest (I)

Review dietary intake with the patient to determine his or her level of adherence to the prescribed diet (I)

Consult with both physician and dietitian (I)

Adjust the diet to the patient's lifestyle (I)

Assist the patient with eating (I)

Communication

Encourage patient self-performance, when possible (I)

Anticipate the patient's need and provide for them (I)

Listen to the patient's concerns, fears, and anxieties (I)

Reduce the patient's anxiety level (I)

Provide knowledge regarding illness and prognosis (ID)

Inform the patient of changes in his or her condition and of the results of laboratory studies (I)

Keep teaching on a simple-to-complex continuum, depending upon the patient (I)

Support the family throughout the patient's hospitalization (I)

Activity

Change the patient's position q2h (I)

Increase positional tolerance by gradually turning and/or positioning the patient in order to provide adequate ventilation (I)

Evaluate the patient for abnormal body movement (I)

Evaluate any alteration in the patient's thought process (I)

Encourage alternative rest and moderate activity periods (I)

Pain

Administer analgesics as prescribed (D)

Estimate the degree of pain expressed (I)

Reassure the patient that the pain will subside or be relieved (I)

Prepare the patient for a painful experience (I)

Discuss possible pain-relieving measures (I)

Ask the patient what makes him or her comfortable (I)

Bibliography

Borg, N., Nikes, D., Stark, J. & Williams, S. *Core curriculum for critical care nursing.* Philadelphia: W. B. Saunders, 1981.

Emanuelson, K. & Densmore, M. *Acute respiratory care.* Bethany, Conn.: Fleschner Publishing Company, 1981.

Wade, J. *Comprehensive respiratory care.* St. Louis: C. V. Mosby, 1982.

Oxygen–Carbon Dioxide Gas Exchange, Crackles

DEFINITION

Crackles, or crepitations, are discontinuous, interrupted explosive sounds with a wide spectrum of frequencies.

ETIOLOGY

Early inspiratory

Emphysema

Chronic bronchitis

Thoracic cage deformities and abnormalities

Carcinoma of the lung

Tuberculosis
Aspiration lung disease
Mid- to late inspiratory
Inhalation or occupational pulmonary disease
Acute pulmonary embolism
Lung abscess
Aspiration lung disease
Wegener's granulomatosis
Early inspiratory–expiratory
Bronchiectasis
Cystic fibrosis
Pulmonary edema
Late inspiratory
Interstitial fibrosis
Sarcoidosis
Nueromuscular disorders
Inhalational or occupational pulmonary disease
Hypersensitivity pneumonitis
Goodpasture's syndrome
Idiopathic pulmonary hemosiderosis
Eosinophilic granuloma
Sickle-cell anemia
Carcinoma of the lung
Bronchial carcinoid
Viral pneumonia
Lung abscess
Pulmonary alveolar proteinosis

DEFINING CHARACTERISTICS

Regulatory Behaviors
Dyspnea
Tachypnea
Fatigue
Cough

Cognitive Behaviors
Restlessness
Anxiety

NURSING RESPONSIBILITIES

Assessment

Assess regulatory behaviors indicative of crackles (I)

Assess cognitive behaviors indicative of crackles (I)

Monitor whether crackles are early, mid- or late inspiratory-expiratory (I)

Assess for the presence of early inspiratory crackles and note their characteristics (I)

> Few in number
>
> Low pitched
>
> Varying in loudness
>
> Not abolished by coughing
>
> Audible at both mouth and lung bases

Assess for the presence of late inspiratory crackles and note their characteristics (I)

> Numerous
>
> Heard over various regions of the lungs, but not at the mouth
>
> Gravity-dependent

Inspect the extremities for edema (I)

Auscultate the heart for abnormal heart sounds (I)

Auscultate the heart for rate, rhythm, and regularity (I)

Palpate arterial pulsations/peripheral pulses for quality and equality (I)

Auscultate the chest to determine the location of the crackles (I)

Inspect the skin for cyanosis (I)

Inspect the patient for shortness of breath or dyspnea (I)

Auscultate the chest for respiratory rate, rhythm, and regularity (I)

Interventions

Fluid

Administer prescribed medications (D)

Administer prescribed IV fluids (D)

Evaluate data from hemodynamic parameters: PAP, PCWP, CVP, and CO (I)

Measure arterial blood pressure and MAP (I)

Evaluate laboratory studies (I)

Evaluate the skin for color, temperature, and presence of diaphoresis (I)

Measure intake, urinary volume, and specific gravity (I)

Aeration

Assist in initiating ventilatory support as ordered (D)

Provide nursing care, such as changing the patient's position, therapy and use aseptic techniques when suctioning (ID)

Establish and maintain a patent airway (I)

Assist the physician with a tracheostomy if necessary (I)

Remove mucous and secretions from the respiratory tract (I)

Encourage the patient to cough, turn, and deep-breathe (I)

Evaluate arterial blood gasses (I)

Evaluate sputum culture data (I)

Nutrition

Encourage the patient to maintain the prescribed diet (I)

Adjust the diet to the patient's lifestyle (I)

Assist the patient with eating (I)

Provide a spiritual support system (I)

Communication

Instruct the patient in the use of the incentive spirometer (I)

Listen to the patient's concerns and fears (I)

Reduce the patient's anxiety level (I)

Prepare the patient for suctioning (I)

Keep teaching on a simple level (I)

Activity

Encourage periods of rest between periods of moderate activity (I)

Change the patient's position q2h (I)

Evaluate for any alterations in the patient's thought process (I)

Pain

Administer prescribed analgesics (D)

Prepare the patient for a painful experience (I)

Ask the patient what makes him or her comfortable (I)

Reassure the patient that the pain will subside or be relieved (I)

Instruct the patient on how to splint an incision or a painful area (I)

Bibliography

Gettrust, K., Ryan, S., & Engleman, D. *Applied nursing diagnosis.* New York: Wiley, 1985.

Kelly, M. *Nursing diagnosis source book.* Norwalk, Conn.: Appleton-Century-Crofts, 1985.

Kim, M. J., McFarland, G., & McLane, A. *Nursing diagnosis.* St. Louis: C. V. Mosby, 1984.

Alteration in Distributive Gas Exchange, Spontaneous Pneumothorax

DEFINITION

When air is introduced into the intrapleural space, causing the negative "pull" to be lost, the lung collapses, resulting in tension, or spontaneous pneumothorax.

ETIOLOGY

Emphysema
Tuberculosis
Congenital cystic disease
Lung abscesses
Cystic fibrosis
Hydatid cyst
Fungus infection
Sarcoma
Asthma
Tuberous sclerosis
Hystiocytosis
Interstitial fibrosis
Lymphangiomyomatosis
Sarcoidosis
Marfan's syndrome
Radiation fibrosis

DEFINING CHARACTERISTICS

Regulatory Behaviors

Chest pain
Anterior in location
Radiation toward sternum, suggesting pneumomediastinum

Dyspnea
Nonproductive cough
Cyanosis
Feeling of constriction in chest
Mediastinal shift
Hypotension

Cognitive Behaviors
Anxiety
Nervousness
Apprehension
Fear
Agitation

NURSING RESPONSIBILITIES

Assessment

Assess regulatory behaviors indicative of spontaneous pneumothorax (I)
Assess cognitive behaviors indicative of spontaneous pneumothorax (I)
Monitor the ECG pattern continuously (I)
Inspect the jugular veins for distension (I)
Auscultate the heart for abnormal heart sounds (I)
Auscultate the chest for pleural friction rub (I)
Palpate the chest for decreased or absent breath sounds (I)
Auscultate the chest for absent breath sounds (I)

Interventions

Fluid

Regulate the IV flow rate (I)
Evaluate the skin for pallor and/or cyanosis (I)
Evaluate laboratory studies (I)
Measure intake, output, and specific gravity (I)

Aeration

Assist the physician with chest-tube insertion (D)
Evaluate with the physician the results of pulmonary function studies and laboratory tests (I)
Reduced lung volume
Reduced compliance

Reduced diffusing capacity

Reduced PaO_2

Review with the physician the patient's chest film (I)

Evaluate the effectiveness of the chest tube, including the amount and color of drainage (I)

Evaluate the patient's breathing pattern for shortness of breath or dyspnea (I)

Auscultate the chest for respiratory rate, rhythm, and regularity (I)

Evaluate the patient's arterial blood gasses (I)

Nutrition

Consult with the dietitian regarding an optimal diet for the patient (I)

Encourage the patient to eat when his or her pulmonary function has stabilized (I)

Communication

Reduce the patient's anxiety level (I)

Provide knowledge regarding the need for a chest tube (I)

Keep instructions simple (I)

Listen to the patient's concerns and fears (I)

Activity

Change the patient's position as needed (I)

Encourage the patient to do passive and active range-of-motion exercises (I)

Prevent infection by using an asceptic/sterile technique when changing IV tubing or the dressing around the chest tube (I)

Evaluate any alteration in the patient's thought process (I)

Pain

Administer prescribed analgesics (D)

Discuss possible pain-relieving measures (I)

Evaluate the type, location, and duration of pain (I)

Bibliography

Harper, R. *A Guide to respiratory care*. Philadelphia: Lippincott, 1981.

Moser, K. & Spragg, R. *Respiratory emergencies*. St. Louis: C. V. Mosby, 1982.

INEFFECTIVE BREATHING PATTERN

Ineffective Breathing Pattern, Alveolar Hypoventilation

DEFINITION

In a state of alveolar hypoventilation, the amount of minute alveolar ventilation is unable to match the body's metabolic rate.

ETIOLOGY

Interference with the neurological conduction of impulses
  Spinal-cord trauma
  Encephalitis
  Tetanus
  Botulism
  Rabies
  Myasthenia gravis
  Pharmacological
    Curare and other myoneural blockers
    Methyl alcohol
    Hypokalemia
    Phenothiazine intoxication
  Paralysis of respiratory muscles
    Muscular dystrophy
    Guillian-Barré syndrome
    Poliomyelitis
  CNS depression
  Pharmacological
    Anesthesia
    Drug overdose
  Disease
    Tumors
    Thrombosis/embolus
    Idiopathic hypoventilation
    Sleep apnea
  Pulmonary conditions
    Chest-wall trauma
    Kyphosoliosis
    Aspiration

> Asthma
> Pulmonary fibrosis
> Pneumonia
> Pulmonary edema
> Pulmonary emboli

DEFINING CHARACTERISTICS

Regulatory Behaviors

Increased work of breathing
Increased minute ventilation
Reduced efficiency of ventilatory muscles
Decreased cardiac output
Tachycardia
Hypotension

Cognitive Behaviors

Altered mental state
Anxiety
Apprehension
Lethargy

NURSING RESPONSIBILITIES

Assessment

Assess regulatory behaviors indicative of alveolar hypo-ventilation (I)
Assess cognitive behaviors indicative of alveolar hypoventilation (I)
Monitor the ECG pattern continuously (I)
Observe the side or therapeutic effects of prescribed medications (I)
Assess the patient's neurological status (I)
Auscultate the heart for abnormal heart sounds (I)
Auscultate the chest for adventitious breath sounds (I)
Auscultate the chest for respiratory rate, rhythm, and regularity (I)

Interventions

Fluid

Administer prescribed medications (D)
Administer prescribed IV fluids (D)

Measure arterial blood pressure and MAP (I)
Measure intake, output, and specific gravity (I)
Evaluate laboratory studies (I)

Aeration
Elevate the head of the bed (I)
Maintain a patent airway (I)
Measure tidal volume and vital capacity (I)
Evaluate the patient's skin for cyanosis (I)
Encourage the patient to cough, turn, and deep-breathe (I)
Provide oxygen at the prescribed flow rate (I)
Provide ventilatory support as needed (I)
Remove mucous and secretions from the respiratory tract (I)

Nutrition
Encourage the patient to maintain the prescribed diet (I)
Adjust the diet to the patient's lifestyle (I)
Assist the patient with eating (I)

Communication
Listen to the patient's concerns, fears, and anxieties (I)
Reduce the patient's anxiety level (I)
Instruct the patient to cough and deep-breathe effectively
    (I)
Instruct the patient to relax accessory muscles (I)
Support the family throughout the patient's hospitaliza-
    tion (I)

Activity
Change the patient's position q2h (I)
Evaluate any alteration in the patient's thought process (I)
Encourage alternative rest and moderate activity periods (I)

Pain
Administer prescribed analgesics (D)
Evaluate the type, location, and duration of pain (I)

Bibliography
Carpenito, L. J. *Handbook of nursing diagnosis.* Philadelphia: Lippin-
    cott, 1984.
Gettrust, K., Ryan, S., & Engleman, D. *Applied nursing diagnosis.* New
    York: Wiley, 1985.

Harper, R. Application of alveolar ventilation physiology. *Dimensions of Critical Care Nursing*, 1(2), 80–86, March–April 1982.

Kelly, M. *Nursing diagnosis souce book.* Norwalk, Conn.: Appleton-Century-Crofts, 1985.

Kim, M.J., McFarland, G., & McLane, A. *Nursing diagnosis.* St. Louis: C. V. Mosby, 1984.

Ineffective Breathing Pattern, Alveolar Hyperventilation

DEFINTION

Alveolar hyperventilation is an increase in alveolar ventilation above the body's metabolic requirements.

ETIOLOGY

Drugs
    Salicylate intoxication
    Respiratory stimulants
    Epinephrine
Metabolic
    Fever
    Hyperthyroidism
    Shock
    Bacteremia
CNS lesions
    Pontine lesions
    Meningitis
    Encephalitis
Pulmonary
    Interstitial lung disease
    Thromboembolism
    Pneumonia
    Atelectasis
    Adult respiratory distress syndrome
    Chronic obstructive pulmonary disease
Psychogenic
    Anxiety
    Pain
    Chronic hyperventilation syndrome

DEFINING CHARACTERISTICS

Regulatory Behaviors
Fatigue
Tachypnea
Dyspnea
Increase tidal volume

Cognitive Behaviors
Nervousness
Anxiety
Irritability

NURSING RESPONSIBILITIES

Assessment
Assess regulatory behaviors indicative of alveolar hyper-ventilation (I)

Assess cognitive behaviors indicative of alveolar hyper-ventilation (I)

Assess situations in which alveolar hyperventilation occur, such as fever, shock, anxiety, or fear (I)

Monitor the ECG pattern continuously (I)

Auscultate the heart for rate, rhythm, and regularity (I)

Auscultate the heart for abnormal heart sounds (I)

Auscultate the chest for adventitous breath sounds (I)

Inspect the skin for cyanosis (I)

Inspect for shortness of breath or dyspnea (I)

Auscultate the chest for respiratory rate, rhythm, and regularity (I)

Percuss the chest for abnormal resonance (I)

Interventions

Fluid
Administer prescribed medications (D)

Administer prescribed IV fluids (D)

Regulate the IV flow rate and check for patency (I)

Measure arterial blood pressure and MAP (I)

Evaluate the skin for color, temperature, and presence of diaphoresis (I)

Measure intake, urinary volume, and specific gravity (I)

Evaluate laboratory studies (I)

Aeration

Provide oxygen at the prescribed flow rate (I)
Encourage the patient to breathe slowly (I)
Reduce meaningless environmental stimuli (I)

Nutrition

Encourage the patient to maintain the prescribed diet (I)
Consult with both physician and dietitian (I)
Adjust the diet to the patient's lifestyle (I)

Communication

Anticipate the patient's needs, and provide for them (I)
Reduce the patient's anxiety level (I)
Encourage patient self-performance, when possible (I)
Listen to the patient's concerns, fears, and anxieties (I)

Activity

Change the patient's position q2h (I)
Evaluate any alterations in the patient's thought process (I)
Encourage alternative rest and moderate activity periods (I)

Pain

Administer analgesics as prescribed (D)
Ask the patient what makes him or her comfortable (I)
Discuss possible pain-relieving measures (I)

Bibliography

Carpenito, L. J. *Handbook of nursing diagnosis.* Philadelphia: Lippincott, 1984.

Gettrust, K., Ryan, S., & Engleman, D. *Applied nursing diagnosis.* New York: Wiley, 1985.

Harper, R. *A guide to respiratory care.* Philadelphia: Lippincott, 1981.

Kelly, M. *Nursing diagnosis source book.* Norwalk, Conn.: Appleton-Century-Crofts, 1985.

Kim, M. J., McFarland, G., & McLane, A. *Nursing diagnosis.* St. Louis: C. V. Mosby, 1984.

Ineffective Breathing Pattern, Dyspnea

DEFINITION

Dyspnea is a subjective feeling of difficult, uncomfortable, or unpleasant breathing.

ETIOLOGY
Obstructive lung disease
  Emphysema
  Chronic bronchitis
  Asthma
  Bronchiectasis
  Cystic fibrosis
Restrictive lung disease
  Interstitial fibrosis
  Sarcoidosis
  Pulmonary edema
  Neuromuscular disorders
  Inhalational or occupational pulmonary diseases
  Hypersensitivity pneumonitis
  Goodpasture's syndrome
  Eosinophilic granuloma
Pulmonary vascular disease
  Acute pulmonary embolism
  Sickle-cell disease
  Recurrent pulmonary thromboembolism
  Primary pulmonary hypertension
  Pulmonary vasocclusive disease
Tumors of the lung, pleura, and medistinum
  Carcinoma of the lung
  Metastatic carcinoma of the lung
  Bronchial adenomas
Infectious disease of the lung
  Bacterial myoplasmal and rickettsial pneumonias
  Viral pneumonia
  Lung abscesses
  Tuberculosis
  Mycoses
Miscellaneous
  Aspiration lung disease
  Pulmonary alveolar proteinosis
  Wegener's granulomatosis

DEFINING CHARACTERISTICS

Regulatory Behaviors
Breathlessness
Fatigue

Cognitive Behaviors
> Sensation of difficult breathing
> Sleep-pattern disturbance
> Anxiety
> Nervousness

NURSING RESPONSIBILITIES

Assessment
> Assess regulatory behaviors indicative of dyspnea (I)
> Assess cognitive behaviors indicative of dyspnea (I)
> Observe the side or therapeutic effects of prescribed medications (I)
> Assess changes in consciousness (I)
> Inspect for trepopnea, which denotes dyspnea occurring in one decubitus position as opposed to the other (I)
> Inspect for platypnea, which refers to dyspnea in the upright position but not in the supine position (I)
> Inspect for orthopnea, which is dyspnea occurring in the supine position but not in the semiupright or upright position (I)
> Inspect for cyanosis (I)
> Inspect for paroxysmal nocturnal dyspnea (I)
> Auscultate the chest for respiratory rate, rhythm, and regularity (I)
> Auscultate the chest for adventitious breath sounds (I)

Interventions

Fluid
> Administer prescribed medications (D)
> Administer prescribed IV fluids (D)
> Measure arterial blood pressure and MAP (I)
> Regulate the IV flow rate and check for patency (I)
> Evaluate data from hemodynamic parameters: PAP, PCWP, CVP, and CO (I)
> Evaluate the skin for color, temperature, and diaphoresis (I)
> Measure intake, output, and specific gravity (I)
> Evaluate data from laboratory studies (I)

Aeration
> Measure tidal volume and vital capacity (I)

Elevate the head of the bed (I)

Maintain a patent airway (I)

Encourage the patient to cough, turn, and deep-breathe (I)

Provide ventilatory support as needed (I)

Remove mucous and secretions from the respiratory tract (I)

Nutrition

Assist the dyspneic patient with eating (I)

Provide periods of rest before eating (I)

Adjust the size of feedings according to the patient's degree of dyspnea (I)

Communication

Instruct the patient to cough and deep-breathe effectively (I)

Instruct the patient to relax accessory muscles (I)

Instruct the patient in the use of pursed-lip breathing (I)

Provide knowledge regarding the causes of dyspnea (I)

Encourage the dyspneic patient to stop smoking (I)

Reduce the patient's anxiety level (I)

Activity

Change the patient's position q2h (I)

Increase positional tolerance by gradually turning and/or positioning the patient in order to provide adequate ventilation (I)

Encourage alternative rest and moderate activity periods (I)

Pain

Administer prescribed analgesics (D)

Evaluate whether or not the patient's pain is due to dyspnea (I)

Reassure the patient that the pain will subside or be relieved (I)

Bibliography

Carpenito, L. J. *Handbook of nursing diagnosis*. Philadelphia: Lippincott, 1984.

Gettrust, K., Ryan, S., & Engleman, D. *Applied nursing diagnosis*. New York: Wiley, 1985.

Glauser, F. *Signs and symptoms in pulmonary medicine*. Philadelphia: Lippincott, 1983.

Kelly, M. *Nursing diagnosis source book.* Norwalk, Conn.: Appleton-
    Century-Crofts, 1985.
Kim, M. J., McFarland, G., & McLane, A. *Nursing diagnosis.* St. Louis:
    C. V. Mosby, 1984.

Ventilation–Perfusion Imbalance

DEFINITION
Ventilation–perfusion imbalance occurs when the lungs will
not perform their function of O_2–CO_2 exchange because
alveolar ventilation and pulmonary capillary blood flow do not
match.

OTHER DEFINITIONS

High Ventilation-Perfusion Ratios
High ventilation–perfusion ratios occur when portions of the
lungs that receive too little perfusion in relation to ventilation
have V–P ratios that are higher than normal.

Low Ventilation-Perfusion Ratios
Low ventilation–perfusion ratios occur when portions of alveoli
receive too little ventilation compared to the amount of blood
flow.

ETIOLOGY
    High V–P ratio
        Pulmonary emboli
        Hyperventilation
    Low V–P ratio
        Pneumonia
        Pulmonary edema
        Atelectasis
        Cystic fibrosis
        Chronic bronchitis
        Adult respiratory distress syndrome

DEFINING CHARACTERISTICS

Regulatory Behaviors
    Tachypnea
    Dyspnea

Cyanosis
Crackles
Hypercarbia
Hypotension
Rusty sputum
Fatigue

Cognitive Behaviors
Decreased sensorium
Anxiety
Fear
Irritability
Lethargy
Apprehension
Confusion

NURSING RESPONSIBILITIES

Assessment
Assess regulatory behaviors indicative of V–P imbalance (I)
Assess cognitive behaviors indicative of V–P imbalance (I)
Monitor the ECG pattern continuously (I)
Assess for potential problems in weaning the patient off
the ventilator (I)
Auscultate the heart for abnormal heart sounds (I)
Auscultate the heart for rate, rhythm, and regularity (I)
Inspect the jugular veins (I)
Auscultate the chest for adventitious breath sounds (I)
Auscultate the chest for respiratory rate, rhythm, and regu-
larity (I)
Inspect for cyanosis (I)
Inspect for shortness of breath or dyspnea (I)

Interventions

Fluid
Provide appropriate IV fluid therapy (D)
Ringer's lactate
Isotonic salt solution
Administer prescribed medications (D)
Antibiotics
Lasix

Edecrin
Digitalis
Methyprednisolone
Measure arterial blood pressure and MAP (I)
Measure intake, urinary volume, and specific gravity (I)
Evaluate the patient's skin for cyanosis (I)
Evaluate data from hemodynamic parameters: PAP, PCWP,
    CVP, SVR, and CO (I)
Evaluate laboratory studies (I)

Aeration

Determine with the physician the degree of anatomic dead
    space, alveolar dead space, functional residual capacity,
    and physiological shunting (D)
Provide humidified oxygen at the prescribed flow rate (D)
Determine with the physician the patient's pulmonary
    vascular resistance (ID)

$$\frac{\text{PA Mean Pressure–LA or PAW Mean Pressure*}}{\text{CO (l/min)}}$$

Evaluate the patient's ventilatory performance with PEEP
    (ID)
Provide pulmonary physical therapy (ID)
Instruct the patient in appropriate breathing to relieve
    dyspnea and to improve ventilatory efficiency, respira-
    tory muscle function, and exercise tolerance (I)
Evaluate arterial blood gasses (I)
Provide ventilatory support as needed (I)

Nutrition

Encourage the patient to eat the prescribed diet (I)
Assist the patient with eating (I)
Provide a spiritual support system (I)

Communication

Reduce the patient's anxiety level (I)
Provide knowledge regarding the use of supportive devices
    (I)

---

*PA = pulmonary artery; LA = left atrial; PAW = pulmonary artery
wedge.

Listen to the patient's concerns regarding his or her illness (I)

Activity

Change the patient's position as necessary (I)

Evaluate any alteration in the patient's thought process (I)

Encourage the patient to perform passive and active range-of-motion exercises (I)

Pain

Administer prescribed analgesics (D)

Evaluate the type, location, and duration of pain (I)

Bibliography

Harper, R. *A guide to respiratory care.* Philadelphia: Lippincott, 1981.

Roberts, S. *Physiological concepts and the critically ill patient.* Englewood Cliffs, N.J.: Prentice-Hall, 1985, pp. 211–244.

INEFFECTIVE AIRWAY CLEARANCE

Ineffective Airway Clearance, Wheezes

DEFINITION

Wheezes are continuous sounds with a musical characteristic and are generated by regular vibrations of the airway walls, which draw their energy from the air flow.

ETIOLOGY

Expiratory

Emphysema

Sarcoidosis

Pulmonary edema

Thoracic cage deformities and abnormalities

Acute pulmonary embolism

Metastatic carcinoma of the lung

Bacterial mycoplasmal and rickettsial pneumonias

Lung abscesses

Tuberculosis

Expiratory–inspiratory

Chronic bronchitis

Asthma

Bronchiectasis

Cystic fibrosis
Inhalational or occupational pulmonary diseases
Hypersensitivity
Carcinoma of the lung
Bronchial carcinoma
Aspiration lung disease
Inspiratory–expiratory
Upper-airway obstruction

DEFINING CHARACTERISTICS

Regulatory Behaviors
Dyspnea
Tachypnea
Cough
Air hunger
Tachycardia
Fatigue

Cognitive Behaviors
Restlessness
Apprehension
Anxiety
Irritability

NURSING RESPONSIBILITIES

Assessment
Assess regulatory behaviors indicative of wheezing (I)
Assess cognitive behaviors indicative of wheezing (I)
Monitor whether wheezes are monophonic or polyphonic (I)
Assess for the presence of monophonic wheezes (I)
Produce single notes
Begin and end at different times during inspiration, expiration, or both
Assess for the presence of polyphonic wheezes (I)
Several musical notes that begin and end simultaneously during expiration
Auscultate the heart for abnormal heart sounds (I)
Auscultate the heart for rate, rhythm, and regularity (I)
Auscultate the chest to determine the timing of wheezes (I)

Palpate the chest for vocal and tactile fremitus (I)
Percuss the chest for abnormal resonance (I)
Auscultate the chest for respiratory rate, rhythm, and regularity (I)

Interventions

Fluid

Administer prescribed medications (D)
Administer prescribed IV fluids (D)
Regulate the IV flow rate and check for patency (I)
Measure intake, output, and specific gravity (I)
Measure arterial blood pressure and MAP (I)
Evaluate laboratory studies (I)

Aeration

Evaluate the patient's skin for cyanosis (I)
Encourage the patient to cough, turn, and deep-breathe (I)
Evaluate the breathing pattern for shortness of breath or dyspnea (I)
Remove mucous and secretions from the respiratory tract (I)
Evaluate arterial blood gasses (I)

Nutrition

Assist the patient with eating (I)
Encourage the patient to maintain the prescribed diet (I)
Consult with both physician and dietitian (I)

Communication

Listen to the patient's concerns, fears, and anxieties (I)
Reduce the patient's anxiety level (I)
Inform the physician of changes in the patient's condition or laboratory studies (I)
Provide knowledge regarding the causes of wheezes (I)

Activity

Change the patient's position q1h (I)
Provide diversional activities (I)
Encourage alternative rest and moderate activity periods (I)

Pain

Administer analgesics as prescribed (D)
Estimate the degree of pain expressed (I)
Discuss possible pain-relieving measures (I)

Bibliography
Carpenito, L. J. *Handbook of nursing diagnosis.* Philadelphia: Lippin-
    cott, 1984.
Gettrust, K., Ryan, S., & Engleman, D. *Applied nursing diagnosis.* New
    York: Wiley, 1985.
Harper, R. *A guide to respiratory care.* Philadelphia: Lippincott, 1981.
Kelly, M. *Nursing diagnosis source book.* Norwalk, Conn.: Appleton-
    Century-Crofts, 1985.
Kim, M. J., McFarland, G., & McLane, A. *Nursing diagnosis.* St. Louis:
    C. V. Mosby, 1984.

Ineffective Airway Clearance, Obstruction

DEFINITION
A state in which the individual experiences ineffective airway
clearance caused by an obstruction to air flow.

ETIOLOGY
    Facial trauma
    Chest trauma
    Pulmonary trauma
    Tenuous mucous
    Bronchiogenic carcinoma
    Asthma
    Bronchitis
    Endotracheal or tracheostomy obstruction

DEFINING CHARACTERISTICS

Regulatory Behaviors
    Shortness of breath
    Dyspnea
    Tachypnea
    Tachycardia
    Cyanosis
    Cough

Cognitive Behaviors
    Anxiety
    Apprehension
    Agitation
    Restlessness
    Panic

NURSING RESPONSIBILITIES

Assessment

Assess regulatory behaviors indicative of airway obstruction (I)

Assess cognitive behaviors indicative of airway obstruction (I)

Monitor the ECG pattern continuously (I)

Observe the side or therapeutic effects of prescribed medications (I)

Auscultate the heart for abnormal heart sounds (I)

Auscultate the chest for adventitious breath sounds (I)

Percuss the chest for resonance, dullness, and flatness (I)

Auscultate the chest for respiratory rate, rhythm, and regularity (I)

Inspect the skin for cyanosis (I)

Interventions

Fluid

Administer prescribed IV fluids (D)

Regulate the IV flow rate (I)

Evaluate the skin for color, temperature, and diaphoresis (I)

Measure blood pressure and MAP (I)

Evaluate data from hemodynamic parameters: PAP, PCWP, CVP, and CO (I)

Evaluate laboratory studies (I)

Measure intake, output, and specific gravity (I)

Aeration

Provide ventilatory support with PEEP (D)

Hyperoxygenate/hyperventilate the patient thoroughly before and after suctioning procedures (ID)

Maintain a patent airway (I)

Remove excess pulmonary secretions using aseptic techniques (I)

Encourage the patient to cough and deep-breathe (I)

Evaluate arterial blood gasses (I)

Evaluate the breathing pattern for shortness of breath or dyspnea (I)

Nutrition

Consult with the dietitian to provide an optimal diet (I)

Adjust the diet to the patient's lifestyle (I)
Assist the patient with eating (I)

Communication
Reduce the patient's anxiety level (I)
Provide knowledge regarding the use of supportive devices (I)
Listen to the patient's concerns (I)
Keep instruction simple (I)

Activity
Change the patient's position frequently to prevent alveolar stasis (I)
Evaluate any alterations in the patient's thought process (I)
Encourage the patient to perform passive and active range-of-motion exercises (I)

Pain
Administer prescribed medications (D)
Evaluate the type, location, and duration of pain (I)
Discuss possible pain-relieving measures (I)

TISSUE PERFUSION, ALTERATION IN
Pulmonary Tissue Perfusion Alteration, Emboli

DEFINITION
Pulmonary emboli are either subacute, which means that they tend to lodge in the distal branches of the pulmonary artery at the periphery of the lung, or they are massive, meaning that one or more of the lobar arteries is involved.

ETIOLOGY
Stasis of blood
    Congestive heart failure
    Atrial fibrillation
    Decreased myocardial contractility
    Prolonged bed rest
Injury to the vascular endothelium
    Local trauma
    Venous disease
    Incision
    Sepsis
    Arteriosclerosis

    Coagualability
        Dehydration
        Sudden elimination of the use of anticoagulants
        Pregnancy
        Estrogen
    Old age
    Cardiopulmonary problems
        Chronic obstructive pulmonary disease
        Cor pulmonale
        History of pulmonary emboli
    Carcinoma
        Pancreas
        Stomach
        Lung

DEFINING CHARACTERISTICS

Regulatory Behaviors

    Dyspnea
    Pleuritic pain
    Tachypnea
    Tachycardia
    Rales
    Splitting S_2
    Edema
    Murmur
    Cyanosis

Cognitive Behaviors

    Anxiety
    Discomfort
    Apprehension
    Restlessness
    Confusion

NURSING RESPONSIBILITIES

Assessment

    Assess regulatory behaviors indicative of pulmonary embolism (I)
    Assess cognitive behaviors indicative of pulmonary embolism (I)

Monitor the ECG pattern continuously (I)

Observe the side or therapeutic effects of prescribed medications (I)

Assess the patient's neurological status (I)

Auscultate the heart for abnormal heart sounds: splitting S_2 (I)

Palpate arterial pulsations/peripheral pulses (I)

Inspect the jugular veins for distension (I)

Auscultate the chest for adventitious breath sounds (I)

Inspect the skin, nail beds, lips, and ear lobes for cyanosis (I)

Auscultate the chest for respiratory rate, rhythm, and regularity (I)

Palpate the chest for the accentuated point of maximum impulse (PMI) (I)

Palpate the chest for evidence of tenderness (I)

Palpate the chest for vocal and/or tactile fremitus (I)

Percuss the chest for resonance, dullness, and flatness (I)

Interventions

Fluid

Administer prescribed medications (D)
   Streptokinase
   Urokinase
   Heparin
   Warfarin
   Persantine
   Aspirin

Assist the physician in measuring pulmonary vascular resistance (PVR) (ID)

Regulate the IV flow rate (I)

Evaluate the skin for color, pallor, or cyanosis (I)

Evaluate the skin for temperature changes and for the presence of diaphoresis (I)

Evaluate data from hemodynamic parameters: PAP, PCWP, CVP, and CO (I)

Measure systemic vascular resistance (SVR) (I)

Measure arterial blood pressure and MAP (I)

Measure intake, urinary volume, and specific gravity (I)

Evaluate laboratory studies: serum enzymes, arterial blood gasses, Lee-White clotting time, activated partial thromboplastin time (APTT), and prothrombin time (PT) (I)

Aeration

Provide humidified oxygen via mask at the prescribed flow rate (D)

Provide ventilatory support with PEEP (D)

Interpret with the physician the patient's chest x-ray (ID)

Evaluate the patient's breathing pattern for dyspnea (I)

Evaluate the patient's arterial blood gasses (I)

Establish and maintain a patent airway (I)

Remove excess pulmonary secretions using aseptic techniques (I)

Encourage the patient to cough and deep-breathe (I)

Nutrition

Provide small, frequent meals for the fatigued and dyspneic patient (I)

Consult with the dietitian to provide an optimal diet (I)

Adjust the diet to the patient's lifestyle (I)

Assist the patient with eating (I)

Communication

Reduce the patient's anxiety level (I)

Provide knowledge regarding diagnostic procedures and supportive devices (I)

Instruct the patient regarding the risk factors leading to deep-vein thrombosis (I)

Instruct the patient regarding the purpose and side effects of anticoagulant therapy (I)

Keep instructions simple (I)

Listen to the patient's concerns, fears, and anxieties (I)

Activity

Ambulate the patient, when possible to decrease the risk of developing a pulmonary embolism (I)

Change the patient's position frequently (I)

Provide antithromboembolic or elastic stockings to promote venous return and to maintain peripheral blood flow (I)

Encourage the patient to perform passive and active range-of-motion exercises (I)

Prevent infections by using aseptic techniques when suctioning or changing tubing (I)

Provide postoperative nursing care, including the use of an umbrella filter and pulmonary embolectomy, for the patient experiencing vena cava interruption (I)

Evaluate any alteration in the patient's thought process (I)

Pain

Administer analgesics as prescribed (D)

Evaluate for the presence of pleuritic pain, characterized by a sharp pain that becomes worse with deep-breathing and coughing (I)

Evaluate for the presence of deep calf pain or the Homan's sign (I)

Discuss possible pain-relieving measures (I)

Ask the patient what makes him or her comfortable (I)

Bibliography

Roberts, S. *Physiological concepts and the critically ill patient.* Englewood Cliffs, N.J.: Prentice-Hall, 1985, pp. 177–210.

INJURY, POTENTIAL FOR

Injury, Chest Trauma

DEFINITION

Chest trauma is defined as a state in which the individual's chest is injured by a blunt or penetrating trauma.

ETIOLOGY

Rib fracture
Flail chest
Sternal fracture
Pneumothorax
Simple pneumothorax
Tension pneumothorax
Open pneumothorax
Hemothorax
Lung injuries
Pulmonary contusion
Laceration of the parenchyma
Injuries to the tracheobronchial tree

Diaphragmatic injuries
Cardiac injuries
   Cardiac contusion
   Penetrating injuries
   Cardiac tamponade
   Injury to the great vessels
   Ruptured branches
   Ruptured esophagus

DEFINING CHARACTERISTICS

Regulatory Behaviors
Pain increasing with inspiration
Shortness of breath
Difficulty breathing
Paradoxic movement of chest
Decreased breath sounds
Tachypnea
Syncope
Hyperesonance on percussion
Hammon's sign
Deviated trachea
Hypotension
Tachycardia
Cyanosis
Distant heart sounds
Ineffective coughing
Chest pain
Hemoptysis
Kussmaul's respiration
Paradoxical pulse
Pleural effusion

Cognitive Behaviors
Restlessness
Agitation
Anxiety
Confusion
Stupor
Coma

NURSING RESPONSIBILITIES

Assessment

Assess regulatory behaviors indicative of chest trauma (I)

Assess cognitive behaviors indicative of chest trauma (I)

Assess airway, breathing, and circulation (I)

Monitor the ECG pattern continuously (I)

Observe the side or therapeutic effects of prescribed medications (I)

Assess intercostal and/or accessory muscle use (I)

Auscultate the heart for rate, rhythm, and regularity (I)

Auscultate the heart for abnormal heart sounds (I)

Palpate peripheral pulses for quality and equality (I)

Auscultate the chest for respiratory rate, rhythm, and regularity (I)

Auscultate the chest for adventitious breath sounds (I)

Auscultate the chest for respiratory stridor (I)

Auscultate the chest for bilateral breath sounds (I)

Inspect for epigastric and supraclavicular indrawing (I)

Inspect for tracheal deviation (I)

Inspect for subcutaneous emphysema (I)

Inspect the chest for sucking sounds (I)

Interventions

Fluid

Administer prescribed IV fluids (D)

Assist the physician with pericardiocentesis if indicated (D)

Administer prescribed medications (ID)

Evaluate arterial blood pressure, CVP, and MAP (I)

Evaluate laboratory studies (I)

Evaluate the patient's skin for color, temperature, and presence of diaphoresis (I)

Measure intake and output (I)

Evaluate wound size and location (I)

Evaluate the jugular veins for distension (I)

Regulate the IV flow rate and check for patency (I)

Aeration

Administer humidified oxygen at the prescribed flow rate (D)

Assist the physician to insert a chest tube into the anterior chest wall if tension pneumothorax is present (D)

Assist the physician with diagnostic procedures (D)
Evaluate for shortness of breath and dyspnea (I)
Evaluate the chest for paradoxical chest movement (I)
Evaluate the tidal volume (I)
Maintain a patent airway (I)
Evaluate arterial blood gasses (I)

Nutrition
NPO

Communication
Reduce the patient's anxiety level (I)
Provide knowledge regarding diagnostic and treatment procedures (I)
Reduce the family's anxiety level by keeping them informed (I)

Activity
Immobilize the patient until the extent of the chest trauma can be evaluated (I)
Evaluate neurological status: pupilary reactions, sensory/motor function, vital signs, and level of consciousness (I)

Pain
Administer analgesics as prescribed (D)
Evaluate the type and intensity of pain (I)

Bibliography

Budassi, S. & Barber, J. *Mosby's manual of emergency care practices and procedures* (2nd ed.). St. Louis: C. V. Mosby, 1984.

Sheehy, S. B., & Barber, J. *Emergency nursing principles and practices*, (2nd ed.). St. Louis: C. V. Mosby, 1985.

NEUROLOGICAL SYSTEM

The critical care nurse begins his or her assessment by inspecting the patient's level and content of consciousness. Furthermore, the nurse uses invasive procedures, such as intracranial pressure monitoring to evaluate changes in intracranial pressure, cerebral tissue perfusion, and the degree of cerebral edema.

CEREBRAL PRESSURE, ALTERATION IN
Intracranial Pressure, Increased

DEFINITION
Intracranial pressure is the pressure exerted by the brain tissue, cerebrospinal fluid, and intravascular blood, which exceeds 200 mg H_2O or 15 mmHg when increased.

ETIOLOGY
Cerebral edema
Cerebral aneurysm
Hemorrhage
    Epidural hematoma
    Subdural hematoma
    Subarachnoid hematoma
CVA
Lesion
Masses
Hyperthermia
Encephalopathy
Hypoxia
Hypercapnia

DEFINING CHARACTERISTICS

Regulatory Behaviors
Headache
Vomiting
Papilledema
    Diplopia
    Nystagmus
    Blurred vision
Pupillary changes
    Pupil dilation
    Pupil construction
    Decreased reaction to light response
Ataxia
Increased systemic blood pressure
Widening pulse pressure
Bradycardia
Changes in respiratory pattern

Change in motor function
Hemiplegia
Hemiparesis
Sensory deterioration
Temperature changes

Cognitive Behaviors
Change in behavior
Inattentiveness
Irritability
Permeability changes
Hallucination
Slurred speech
Change in level of consciousness
Forgetfulness
Memory impairment
Disorientation
Confusion
Sleepiness
Lethargy

NURSING RESPONSIBILITIES

Assessment
Assess regulatory behaviors indicative of increased intracranial pressure (I)
Assess cognitive behaviors indicative of increased intracranial pressure (I)
Monitor the ECG pattern continuously (I)
Assess the patient's neurological status: level of consciousness, pupils, sensory/motor function, and vital signs (I)
Monitor for precipitating factors that further increase intracranial pressure: hypoxia, hypercapnia, fever, hypotension, hypertension, or shock (I)
Monitor intracranial pressure via intravascular, subarachnoid, or epidural devices (I)
Auscultate the heart for abnormal heart sounds (I)
Auscultate the heart for rate, rhythm, and regularity (I)
Inspect the jugular veins for distension (I)
Palpate for arterial pulsations/peripheral pulses (I)

Auscultate the chest for respiratory rate, rhythm, and regularity (I)

Auscultate the chest for normal and abnormal breath sounds (I)

Inspect for dyspnea (I)

Interventions

Fluid

Limit fluid intake from 900 cc to 2500 cc/24 hr (D)

Administer appropriate IV fluids (D)

  Mannitol (Osmitol)

    1.5 to 2 g/kg of body weight

  Glucose

    50% glucose in 50 to 100 cc fluid

Administer prescribed medications (D)

  Edecrin

  Lasix

  Decadron

  Solumedrol

  Pentobarbital sodium

  Dilantin

Evaluate data from continuous intracranial monitoring (I)

  Ventricular pressure (normal 15 mmHg)

  Intracranial pressure (ICP) waveforms

    A waves: plateau or Lundenberg waves seen in advanced stages of increased ICP > 20 mmHg

    B waves: sharp, rhythmic oscillations seen in relationship to fluctuations in respiratory pattern, such as Cheyne-Stokes

    C waves: Traube-Hering-Mayer waves that relate to the normal changes in systemic arterial pressure (SAP)

Calculate cerebral perfusion pressure (CPP) (I)

Regulate the IV flow rate and check for patency (I)

Evaluate the effect of barbiturate coma on intracranial pressure (I)

Measure arterial blood pressure and MAP (I)

Evaluate data from hemodynamic parameters: PAP, PCWP, CVP, SVR, and CO (I)

Measure intake and output (I)

Evaluate specific factors indicating that the barbiturate can
be discontinued and report the findings to the physician (I)
ICP < 15 torr for 24 to 72 hr
Systolic blood pressure < 90 torr, despite the use of
dopamine
Lack of ICP response
Progressive neurological impairment
Abolition of need for vasodilator therapy to reduce
systolic blood pressure below 160 torr
Cardiac arrest
Measure the amount and color of ventricular drainage (I)
Evaluate the patient's temperature (I)
Evaluate laboratory studies: CBC, PT, PTT, platelets, elec-
trolytes, BUN, creatinine, glucose, and serum osmolarity
(I)

Aeration
Hyperinflate the lung with 100% oxygen for 1 min prior to
suctioning (D)
Administer oxygen at the prescribed percentage (D)
Maintain adequate ventilation through the use of continuous
ventilatory support (D)
Suction as necessary, for no more than 15 sec (I)
Evaluate arterial blood gasses for hypoxemia or hypercapnia
(I)
Maintain a patent airway (I)
Instruct the conscious patient not to cough or strain with
stool (I)
Provide aseptic tracheostomy care (I)

Nutrition
Assist the patient with his or her diet (I)
Withhold food and drink from the patient experiencing
nausea or vomiting (I)
Provide oral hygiene (I)

Communication
Evaluate the patient's communication pattern (I)
Inform the physician of any changes in the patient's condi-
tion (I)
Reduce the patient's anxiety level (I)

Provide knowledge regarding invasive or diagnostic procedures (I)

Listen to the patient's concerns (I)

Provide alternative means of communication for the patient with an endotracheal tube or tracheostomy (I)

Reduce the family's anxiety level (I)

Encourage the patient to strive toward realistic goals (I)

Activity

Maintain the patient on complete bed rest (I)

Place the patient in the semi-Fowler's position, with the head elevated to 30 degrees (I)

Reposition and turn the patient q2h if neurologically feasible (I)

Provide skin care with position change (I)

Assist the patient in moving up in bed (I)

Inspect the site of intracranial monitoring for redness or drainage (I)

Change the dressing around the intracranial monitoring device (I)

Encourage passive range-of-motion exercises (I)

Evaluate for abnormal physical activity or movement (I)

Support the patient through seizure activity (I)

Pain

Evaluate the patient's perception of and/or sensitivity to pain (I)

Evaluate the type, location, and duration of pain (I)

Discuss possible pain-relieving measures (I)

Prepare the patient for a painful experience (I)

Reassure the patient that the pain will subside or be relieved (I)

Reduce physical discomforts that could interfere with cognitive functions (I)

Bibliography

Gettrust, K., Ryan, S., & Engleman, D. *Applied nursing diagnosis.* New York: Wiley, 1985.

Hickey, J. *Clinical practice of neurological and neurosurgical nursing.* Philadelphia: Lippincott, 1981.

Johanson, B., Dungca, C., Hoffmeister, D., & Wells, S. *Standards for critical care* (2nd ed.). St. Louis: C. V. Mosby, 1985.

Roberts, S. *Physiological concepts and the critically ill patient.* Englewood Cliffs, N.J.: Prentice-Hall, 1985, pp. 448–498.

Rutkowski-Conway Long, B. *Neurological and neurosurgical nursing.* St. Louis: C. V. Mosby, 1982.

CENTRAL NERVOUS SYSTEM, ALTERATION IN
Ineffective Neuron Activity, Seizure

DEFINITION

A seizure is defined as a sudden, excessive, disorderly discharge of cerebral neurons, which produces an intermittent derangement of the nervous system.

ETIOLOGY

Infection
   Meningitis
   Encephalitis
Space-occupying lesions
   Tumors
   Hematomas
   Abscesses
   Cystic masses
Hemorrhage into the cranial cavity
Head trauma
Neurological damage from deficient supplies
   Anoxia
   Hypoglycemia
Cerebral edema
Degenerative disorders
Metrazol
Alcohol
   Intoxication
   Abrupt withdrawal
Fever

DEFINING CHARACTERISTICS

Regulatory Behaviors
   Tonus
   Clonus

Aura
    Visual
    Auditory
    Gustatory
    Dizziness
    Numbness of body part
Headache

Cognitive Behaviors
    Depression
    Anxiety
    Apprehension
      Loss of control
    Lassitude

NURSING RESPONSIBILITIES

Assessment

Assess regulatory behaviors associated with seizure activity (I)

Assess cognitive behaviors associated with seizure activity (I)

Monitor the ECG pattern continuously (I)

Assess prehospital factors contributing to seizure activity (I)

Assess the patient's neurological status: pupillary reactions, sensory/motor function, level of consciousness, and vital signs (I)

Assess the specific type of seizure activity: grand mal, petit mal, akinetic, myoclonic, psychomotor, visual, or Jacksonian (I)

Auscultate the heart for rate, rhythm, and regularity (I)

Auscultate the chest for respiratory rate, rhythm, and regularity (I)

Inspect for cyanosis (I)

Interventions

Fluid

Administer prescribed medications (D)

Administer prescribed IV fluids (I)

Measure arterial blood pressure and MAP (I)

Measure intake and output (I)

Aeration
> Administer oxygen at the prescribed percentage and flow rate (D)
> Maintain patent airway during and after seizure (I)
> Remove excess secretions using aseptic technique (I)
> Evaluate the patient's breathing pattern for shortness of breath or dyspnea (I)

Nutrition
> Withhold food and drink from the patient experiencing seizure (I)
> Assist the patient with his or her diet (I)

Communication
> Inform the physician of the type and length of the patient's seizure (I)
> Provide knowledge regarding the possible causes of seizure activity (I)
> Reduce the family's anxiety regarding seizure activity (I)
> Listen to the patient's concerns regarding the seizure experience (I)

Activity
> Provide seizure precautions (I)
> Protect the patient from self-injury during the seizure (I)
> Change the patient's position as necessary (I)
> Encourage passive range-of-motion exercises (I)
> Evaluate for abnormal physical activity or movement (I)
> Support the patient through the seizure activity (I)
> Provide frequent rest periods (I)

Pain
> Administer prescribed medications (D)
> Prepare the patient for a painful experience (I)
> Evaluate the type, location, and duration of pain (I)

Bibliography

Hickey, J. *Clinical practice of neurological and neurosurgical nursing.* Philadelphia: Lippincott, 1981.

Johanson, B., Dungca, C., Hoffmeister, D., & Wells, S. *Standards for critical care* (2nd ed.). St. Louis: C. V. Mosby, 1985.

Roberts, S. *Physiological concepts and the critically ill patient.* Englewood Cliffs, N.J.: Prentice-Hall, 1985, pp. 448–498.

Rutkowski-Conway Long, B. *Neurological and neurosurgical nursing.*
St. Louis: C. V. Mosby, 1982.

Extracellular Fluid-Volume Excess, Cerebral Edema

DEFINITION
Cerebral edema results from injury to the cerebral tissue or from certain physiological conditions.

ETIOLOGY
Trauma
    Confusion
    Surgery
Hematoma
    Epidural
    Subdural
    Subarachnoid
Meningitis
Brain tumor
Infarction
Fever
Hypertension

DEFINING CHARACTERISTICS
Regulatory Behaviors
Reduced cerebral blood flow
Increased CPP
Increased cerebral spinal fluid pressure
Reduced capillary blood flow
Increased CVR
Increased intracranial pressure
Bradycardia
Pupillary changes
Sensory/motor changes
Headache
Vomiting
Increased SBP
Widening pulse pressure
Change in respiratory pattern

Cognitive Behaviors
Irritability
Forgetfulness
Memory impairment
Disorientation
Confusion
Lethargy

NURSING RESPONSIBILITIES

Assessment

Assess regulatory behaviors reflecting cerebral edema (I)
Assess cognitive behaviors reflecting cerebral edema (I)
Monitor the ECG pattern continuously (I)
Assess the patient's neurological status: pupillary changes, level of consciousness, sensory/motor function, and vital signs (I)
Monitor intracranial pressure if necessary (I)
Inspect the jugular veins (I)
Auscultate the chest for respiratory rate, rhythm, and regularity (I)
Inspect for cyanosis (I)

Interventions

Fluid

Administer appropriate IV fluids (D)
Administer prescribed medications (D)
Evaluate data from continuous intrancranial monitoring, if used (I)
Regulate the IV flow rate and check for patency (I)
Measure intake and output (I)
Measure blood pressure and MAP (I)
Evaluate data from hemodynamic parameters: PAP, PCWP, CVP, and CO (I)

Aeration

Administer oxygen at the prescribed percentage and flow rate (D)
Evaluate the patient's breathing for shortness of breath or dyspnea (I)
Maintain a patent airway (I)

Nutrition

Assist the patient with his or her diet (I)

Provide oral hygiene (I)

Communication

Inform the physician of changes in the patient's intracranial pressure (I)

Reduce the patient's anxiety level (I)

Reassure the patient regarding his or her condition (I)

Activity

Maintain the patient on complete bed rest until intracranial pressure decreases (I)

Place the patient in semi-Fowler's position, with the head elevated to 30 degrees (I)

Change the patient's position, if realistic, q2h (I)

Evaluate for abnormal physical activity or movement (I)

Pain

Administer prescribed medications (D)

Evaluate the type, location, and duration of pain (I)

Bibliography

Hickey, J. *Clinical practice of neurological and neurosurgical nursing.* Philadelphia: Lippincott, 1981.

Johanson, B., Dungca, C., Hoffmeister, D., & Wells, S. *Standards for critical care* (2nd ed.). St. Louis: C. V. Mosby, 1985.

Roberts, S. *Physiological concepts and the critically ill patient.* Englewood Cliffs, N.J.: Prentice-Hall, 1985, p. 448–498.

Rutkowski-Conway Long, B. *Neurological and neurosurgical nursing.* St. Louis: C. V. Mosby, 1982.

Thought Process, Altered, Loss of Consciousness

DEFINITION

Loss of consciousness is a condition in which there is reduced mental function and altered wakefulness.

ETIOLOGY

Coma

Cerebral trauma

Hemorrhage
   Epidural
   Subdural
   Subarachnoid
CVA
Masses
Lesions

DEFINING CHARACTERISTICS

Regulatory Behaviors
Reduced auditory stimuli
Reduced pain response
   Purposeful response
   Nonpurposeful response
   Unresponsive
Coma

Cognitive Behaviors
Confusion
Delirium
Obtundation
Stupor

NURSING RESPONSIBILITIES

Assessment
Assess regulatory behaviors indicative of loss of consciousness (I)
Assess cognitive behaviors indicative of loss of consciousness (I)
Monitor the ECG pattern continuously (I)
Assess other components of neurological examination: pupillary changes, sensory/motor function, and vital signs (I)
Observe the side or therapeutic effects of prescribed medications (I)
Auscultate the heart for rate, rhythm, and regularity (I)
Inspect the jugular veins (I)
Auscultate the chest for adventitious breath sounds (I)
Inspect for cyanosis (I)

Interventions

Fluid

Administer prescribed IV fluids (D)

Administer prescribed medications (D)

Measure intake and output (D)

Evaluate the patient's level of consciousness by using Glasgow Coma Scale (I)

Evaluate the patient's pupillary reactions and sensory/motor status by using the Glasgow Coma Scale (I)

Evaluate data from laboratory studies (I)

Evaluate data from continuous intracranial monitoring, if used (I)

Aeration

Administer oxygen at the prescribed percentage and flow rate (D)

Suction as necessary, for no more than 15 sec (I)

Maintain a patent airway for the unconscious patient (I)

Evaluate the patient's breathing pattern for dyspnea (I)

Evaluate arterial blood gasses (I)

Nutrition

NPO

Communication

Reduce the family's anxiety level (I)

Listen to the family's concerns and fears (I)

Inform the physician of any changes in the patient's consciousness level (I)

Activity

Change the patient's position q2h (I)

Provide skin care with position change (I)

Evaluate for the presence of decerebrate or decortical activity (I)

Pain

Evaluate the patient's sensitivity to pain (I)

Bibliography

Hickey, J. *Clinical practice of neurological and neurosurgical nursing.* Philadelphia: Lippincott, 1981.

Roberts, S. *Physiological concepts and the critically ill patient.* Engle-
    wood Cliffs, N.J.: Prentice-Hall, 1985, pp. 448-498.
Rutkowski-Conway Long, B. *Neurological and neurosurgical nursing.*
    St. Louis: C. V. Mosby, 1982.

THERMOREGULATION, ALTERATION IN
Hyperthermia

DEFINITION
An elevation of body temperature above the normal range
(99.4°F or greater), usually due to disease (Geels, 1985).

ETIOLOGY
  Excessive exercise
  CNS infection
  Immunologic disorders
      Collagen disease
      Drug fevers
  Dehydration
  Hematopoietic disorders
  Neoplastic disorders
      Hodgkins' disease
      Leukemia
  Subarachnoid hemorrhage
  Lesion of the hypothalamus
  Traction on the hypothalamus or brain stem
  Bacterial endocarditis
  Pneumonia
  Pulmonary embolism
  Myocardial infarction
  CVA
  Malignant hypertension due to anesthesia and other pharma-
      cologic agents
  Hypermetabolic disorders ("thyroid crisis")

DEFINING CHARACTERISTICS

Regulatory Behaviors
  Chills
  Increased respiratory rate

Increased heart rate
Diaphoresis/sweating
Peripheral vasodilatation

Cognitive Behaviors
Confusion

NURSING INTERVENTIONS

Assessment
Inspect the skin for petechiae (I)
Palpate the abdomen for enlarged liver or spleen (I)
Palpate the lymph nodes for evidence of tenderness or en-
largement, indicating infection (I)
Monitor alterations in temperature patterns (I) such as:
    Intermittent: The temperature is elevated for periods of
        time but falls to normal at the same time each day
    Remittent: The temperature rises and falls each day but
        does not return to normal
    Sustained: The temperature is elevated with less than a
        0.5°F variation during a 24-hour period
    Relapsing: Short, febrile periods are interspersed with
        longer periods of normal temperature
    Hectic or septic: A fever in which there are wide varia-
        tions of at least 2.5°F each day
Weigh patient daily (I)
Inspect the skin for dehydration (I)
Assess regulatory behaviors indicative of hyperthermia (I)
Monitor the ECG pattern continuously (I)
Assess the patient's level of consciousness (I)
Auscultate the heart for abnormal heart sounds (I)
Auscultate the heart for rate, rhythm, and regularity (I)
Auscultate the chest for adventitious breath sounds (I)
Auscultate the chest for respiratory rate, rhythm, and regu-
larity (I)
Inspect for dyspnea (I)
Palpate the chest for vocal or tactile fremitus (I)

Interventions

Fluid
Administer prescribed medications, such as Aspirin or
acetaminophen (Tylenol), as ordered or as needed (D)

Provide fluid and electrolyte replacement as ordered (D)

Regulate the IV rate and check for patency (I)

Evaluate laboratory studies: serum electrolyte, hematocrit, hemaglobin, BUN, creatine, and blood gasses (I)

Measure arterial blood pressure (I)

Evaluate data from hemodynamic parameters: PAP, PCWP, CVP, and CO (I)

Aeration

Encourage the patient to cough, turn, and deep-breathe (I)

Establish and maintain a patent airway (I)

Suction as necessary via tracheostomy or endotracheal tube (I)

Reduce meaningless environmental noise, when possible (I)

Nutrition

Encourage the patient to eat high-protein foods (I)

Consult with the dietitian regarding suggestions about the palatability and nutritional value of various foods (I)

Assist the patient with his or her diet if necessary (I)

Communication

Provide knowledge regarding medications taken to reduce the patient's temperature (I)

Provide knowledge regarding the purpose behind cooling measures to reduce the patient's temperature (I)

Inform the patient of the record being kept of his or her temperature at regular intervals (I)

Reduce the patient's anxiety level regarding any fluctuations in his or her temperature (I)

Activity

Apply a hypothermia blanket to reduce the patient's temperature (I)

Change the patient's position q2h (I)

Orient the patient as to time, place, and location should confusion occur (I)

Encourage ambulation as soon as the patient's temperature subsides and his or her condition allows increased physical activity (I)

Pain

Administer prescribed analgesics (D)

Evaluate the type, location, and duration of pain (I)
Ask the patient what makes him/her comfortable (I)

Bibliography

Geels, W. In Jacobs, M. & Geels, W., (eds.) *Fever. Signs and Symptoms in Nursing.* Philadelphia: Lippincott, 1985, pp. 291-305.

Hypothermia

DEFINITION

Hypothermia is defined as a body temperature below the normal physiologic level of $37°C$ or $98.6°F$ (Soukup, 1981).

ETIOLOGY

Accidental hypothermia
 Drowning
 Exposure to cold temperature
 Individuals receiving rapid infusion of refrigerated bank
  blood or intravenous solution
 Drugs interfering with the thermal regulatory apparatus
  Alcohol
  Phenothiazides
  Chlorpromazine
  Carbon monoxide
 Secondary to diseases such as
  Hypoglycemia
  Adrenal insufficiency
  Hypopituitarism
  Myxedema
Elective hypothermia
 Cardiovascular surgery
 Neurosurgery
 Febrile multra trauma
 Acute cerebral ischemia
 Burn insults
 Thyroid crisis

DEFINING CHARACTERISTICS

Regulatory Behaviors
 Reduced oxygen consumption

Arrhythmias
  Bradycardia
  Atrial fibrillation
  Atrioventricular blocks
  Premature ventricular contraction
  Ventricular tachycardia
  Muscle tremor artifact
Decreased respiration
Decreased blood pressure
Decreased venous and cerebrospinal fluid pressures
Decreased cerebral blood flow (6% for every degree that the centigrade temperature is reduced below normal)
Oxygen-hemoglobin dissociation curve is shifted to the left
Reduced carbon dioxide concentration

Cognitive Behaviors
  Confusion

NURSING RESPONSIBILITIES

Assessment
  Assess regulatory behaviors indicative of hypothermia (I)
  Assess cognitive behaviors indicative of hypothermia (I)
  Monitor the ECG pattern continuously (I)
  Monitor situations or factors contributing to hypothermia (I)
  Auscultate the heart for abnormal heart sounds (I)
  Inspect for the presence of edema secondary to increased cell permeability (I)
  Monitor the patient's neurological status: pupils, vital signs, sensory-motor function, and level of consciousness (I)
  Assess the skin for discoloration or hardness (I)
  Auscultate the chest for adventitious breath sounds (I)
  Auscultate the chest for respiratory rate, rhythm, and regularity (I)

Interventions

Fluid
  Measure fluid intake so as to prevent fluid imbalance (I)

Measure urinary output as evidence of oliguria or anuria (I)

Administer prescribed medications to control shivering (Curare, succinylcholine, or chlorpromazine) (D)

Evaluate the rectal temperature during rewarming phase (I)

Measure arterial blood pressure (I)

Evaluate data from hemodynamic parameters: PAP, PCWP, CVP, SVR, and CO (I)

Regulate the IV flow rate and check for patency (I)

Aeration

Eliminate or control negative environmental stimuli, such as noise, light, or interruptions (I)

Evaluate arterial blood gasses for evidence of metabolic acidosis (I)

Establish and maintain a patent airway (I)

Nutrition

Assist the patient with his or her diet (I)

Adjust the diet to the person's lifestyle (I)

Communication

Listen to the patient's verbalization of discomfort during intentional hypothermia (I)

Provide knowledge regarding planned hypothermia (I)

Reduce the patient's anxiety level (I)

Reduce the demand for cognitive functioning when the person is ill or fatigued (I)

Activity

Evaluate intracranial pressure in patients with an intracranial monitoring device (I)

Provide gradual rewarming of the patient when appropriate, taking care to prevent vasodilatation, which could lead to hypotension (I)

Massage the skin to prevent any alteration in skin integrity (I)

Pain

Administer prescribed analgesics (D)

Evaluate the type, location, and duration of pain (I)

Bibliography

Rutkowski-Conway Long, B. *Neurological and Neurosurgical Nursing*, 8th Edition. St. Louis: C. V. Mosby, 1982.

Soukup, Sr. M. Hypothermia. In Kinney, M., Dear, C., Packa, D., and Voorman, D. *AACN's Clinical Reference For Clinical Care Nursing*. (eds.). New York: McGraw-Hill, 1981, pp. 991–996.

TISSUE PERFUSION, ALTERATION IN
Cerebral Tissue Perfusion, Decreased

DEFINITION
Decreased cerebral tissue perfusion implies that perfusion through the brain is less than 50 to 55 ml/100 g of brain/min.

ETIOLOGY
    Reduced cardiac output
    Transient ischemic attack
    Cerebral arterial spasm
    Decreased cerebral perfusion pressure
    Increased SAP
    Increased intracranial pressure

DEFINING CHARACTERISTICS

Regulatory Behaviors
    Numbing of extremities
    Dizziness
    Hemiparesis
    Tingling
    Pain
    Headache
    Altered speech
    Coma

Cognitive Behaviors
    Confusion

Irritability
Anxiety
Stupor
Unconsciousness

NURSING RESPONSIBILITIES

Assessment

Assess regulatory behaviors indicative of decreased cerebral tissue perfusion (I)

Assess cognitive behaviors indicative of decreased cerebral tissue perfusion (I)

Monitor the ECG pattern continuously (I)

Assess the patient's neurological status: level of consciousness, pupillary changes, sensory/motor changes, and vital signs (I)

Monitor intracranial pressure (I)

Auscultate the heart for rate, rhythm, and regularity (I)

Auscultate the chest for abnormal breath sounds (I)

Auscultate the chest for adventitious breath sounds (I)

Interventions

Fluid

Administer prescribed medications (D)

Administer prescribed IV fluids (D)

Measure cerebral blood flow (I)

Cerebral blood flow = MAP − ICP

Evaluate CPR (I)

Perfusion pressure = MAP

Measure blood pressure and MAP (I)

Measure intake, urinary volume, and specific gravity (I)

Evaluate laboratory studies (I)

Aeration

Administer oxygen at the prescribed percentage and flow rate (D)

Maintain a patent airway (I)

Evaluate breathing pattern for shortness of breath or dyspnea (I)

Evaluate the patient's skin for cyanosis (I)

Nutrition
   Encourage the patient to maintain the prescribed diet (I)
   Assist the patient with his or her diet (I)

Communication
   Evaluate the patient's communication pattern (I)
   Reduce the patient's anxiety level (I)
   Listen to the patient's concerns and fears (I)
   Inform the physician of any changes in the patient's condi-
      tion (I)

Activity
   Change the patient's position as needed (I)
   Evaluate the patient for abnormal physical activity or move-
      ment (I)
   Evaluate any alterations in the patient's thought process (I)
   Encourage alternative rest and moderate activity periods (I)

Pain
   Evaluate the patient's perception of and/or sensitivity to
      pain (I)
   Evaluate the type, location, and duration of pain (I)

Bibliography

Johanson, B., Dungca, C., Hoffmeister, D., & Wells, S. *Standards for
   critical care.* St. Louis: C. V. Mosby, 1985.
Roberts, S. *Physiological concepts and the critically ill patient.* Englewood Cliffs, N.J.: Prentice-Hall, 1985, pp. 448–498.

Cerebral Perfusion, Obstructed, Thromboembolism

DEFINITION
Thromboembolism occurs when atheroma obstructs the internal carotid artery, middle cerebral artery, anterior cerebral
artery, vertebral–basilar circulatory system, basilar artery, or
posterior cerebral artery.

ETIOLOGY
   Artery-to-artery embolism
   Cardiac emboli
   Lacunar infarction

Hemodynamic factors
Nonarteriosclerotic vasculopathies
Mechanical interference with arteries
Coagulation abnormalities
Thrombocytosis
Cerebral venous and sinus thrombosis

DEFINING CHARACTERISTICS

Regulatory Behaviors
Weakness
Sensory disturbance of face, arm, or leg
Dysphasia
Hemiplegia
Vertigo
Dysopia
Headache
Incontinence

Cognitive Behaviors
Confusion
Combativeness
Irritability
Apprehension
Lassitude
Stupor
Coma

NURSING RESPONSIBILITIES

Assessment
Assess regulatory behaviors indicative of cerebral thrombo-
    embolism (I)
Assess cognitive behaviors indicative of cerebral thrombo-
    embolism (I)
Monitor the ECG pattern continuously (I)
Assess the patient's neurological status: level of conscious-
    ness, sensory/motor changes, pupillary changes, and vital
    signs (I)
Auscultate the heart for rate, rhythm, and regularity (I)
Palpate for arterial pulsations/peripheral pulses (I)
Evaluate skin for cyanosis (I)

Interventions

Fluid

Administer prescribed medications (D)

Administer prescribed IV fluids (D)

Regulate the IV flow rate and check for patency (I)

Measure arterial blood pressure and MAP (I)

Measure intake and output (I)

Evaluate the patient's skin for color, temperature, and presence of diaphoresis (I)

Aeration

Maintain a patent airway (I)

Evaluate the patient's breathing pattern for shortness of breath, dyspnea, or Cheyne-Stokes breathing (I)

Evaluate arterial blood gasses (I)

Administer oxygen at the prescribed percentage and flow rate (D)

Suction as necessary to remove excess pulmonary secretions (I)

Nutrition

Encourage the patient to maintain the prescribed diet (I)

Assist the patient with his or her diet (I)

Encourage a significant other to eat with the patient (I)

Communication

Evaluate the patient's communication pattern (I)

Inform the physician of any changes in the patient's condition (I)

Listen to the patient's concerns (I)

Reduce the family's anxiety level (I)

Encourage the patient to strive toward realistic goals (I)

Activity

Change the patient's position q2h (I)

Encourage passive range-of-motion exercises to the nonaffected extremity (I)

Exercise the affected extremity to maintain muscle tone (I)

Encourage the patient to be as independent as physically realistic (I)

Evaluate the degree of abnormal physical activity or movement (I)

Evaluate any alterations in thought process (I)

Pain

Administer prescribed analgesics (D)

Reduce physical discomfort that could interfere with cognitive function (I)

Reassure the patient that pain will subside or be relieved (I)

Bibliography

Hickey, J. *Clinical practice of neurological and neurosurgical nursing.* Philadelphia: Lippincott, 1981.

Rutkowski-Conway Long, B. *Neurological and neurosurgical nursing.* St. Louis: C. V. Mosby, 1982.

Wyngaarden, J. & Smith, L. *Cecil textbook of medicine* (17th ed.). Philadelphia: W. B. Saunders, 1985.

Vasodilatation of the Vascular Bed, Neurogenic Shock

DEFINITION

In neurogenic shock, there is massive vasodilatation, with subsequent decreased blood pressure, decreased venous return, and decreased cardiac output.

ETIOLOGY

Deep anesthesia

Insulin shock

Spinal anesthesia

Brain damage

Concussions

Contusion of basal areas of brain

Prolonged ischemia of medulla oblongata

Fainting

DEFINING CHARACTERISTICS

Regulatory Behaviors

Hypotension

Tachycardia

Edema

Dizziness
Hypoxia
Decreased CVP
Decreased CO
Oliguria
Arrhythmias
Weakness

Cognitive Behaviors
Anxiety
Apprehension
Irritability
Nervousness
Lassitude
Stupor

NURSING RESPONSIBILITIES

Assessment
Assess regulatory behaviors indicative of neurogenic shock (I)
Assess cognitive behaviors indicative of neurogenic shock (I)
Monitor situations in which neurogenic shock may occur (I)
Monitor the ECG pattern continuously (I)
Observe the side or therapeutic effects of prescribed medications (I)
Auscultate the heart for abnormal heart sounds (I)
Auscultate the chest for respiratory rate, rhythm, and regularity (I)
Auscultate the chest for adventitious breath sounds (I)

Interventions

Fluid
Administer prescribed IV fluids (D)
Administer prescribed medications (D)
Measure blood pressure and MAP (I)
Measure intake and urinary volume (I)
Evaluate the quality and equality of peripheral pulses (I)
Evaluate the skin for color, temperature, and presence of diaphoresis (I)

Aeration

Administer oxygen at the prescribed percentage and flow rate (D)

Evaluate arterial blood gasses (I)

Evaluate the skin for pallor or cyanosis (I)

Nutrition

Encourage the patient to maintain the prescribed diet (I)

Assist the patient with his or her diet (I)

Communication

Listen to the patient's concerns (I)

Provide knowledge regarding the cause of neurogenic shock (I)

When realistic, inform the patient that the problem will subside (I)

Reduce the patient's anxiety level (I)

Activity

Change the patient's position q2h or as necessary (I)

Evaluate any alteration in the patient's thought process (I)

Evaluate for abnormal physical activity or movement (I)

Provide skin care with position change (I)

Pain

Evaluate the type, location, and duration of pain (I)

Discuss possible pain-relieving measures (I)

Bibliography

Bordicks, K. *Patterns of shock implications for nursing care* (2nd ed.). New York: Macmillan, 1980.

Speech Pattern, Altered, Aphasia

DEFINITION

The terms aphasia and dysphasia describe an impairment or loss of language function as a result of damage to the specific language areas of the cerebrum.

ETIOLOGY
Lesions of dominant posterior superior temporal gyrus
   Destroy the capacity to recognize the sensory symbols
      of language or to transform inner thoughts into mean-
      ingful words
         Wernicke's aphasia
Lesion into premotor cortex
   Disturbance in the output of either spontaneous or com-
      manded speech and writing
         Broca's aphasia
Lesion in primary speech area
   Loss of all aspects of language function
      Global aphasia
Lesion of the angular gyrus
   Rambling, lengthy, empty, and poorly focused speech
      Anomic aphasia
Vascular lesions of the left frontal lobe
   Inability to speak
      Mutism

DEFINING CHARACTERISTICS

Regulatory Behaviors
   Right hemiparesis, worse in arm
   Sensory loss in right arm

Cognitive Behaviors
   Depressed mood
   Euphoria
   Paranoia
   Flat effect

NURSING RESPONSIBILITIES

Assessment
   Assess regulatory behaviors indicative of aphasia (I)
   Assess cognitive behaviors indicative of aphasia (I)
   Assess the patient's neurological status: loss of conscious-
      ness, pupillary changes, sensory/motor, and vital signs (I)
   Assess the type of speech-pattern alteration (I)
   Auscultate the heart for rate, rhythm, and regularity (I)

Auscultate the chest for abnormal breath sounds (I)
Auscultate the chest for adventitious breath sounds (I)

Interventions

Fluid

Administer prescribed medications (D)
Administer prescribed IV fluids (D)
Measure blood pressure and MAP (I)
Measure intake and output (I)
Evaluate the patient's skin for color, temperature, and presence of diaphoresis (I)

Aeration

Suction the patient as necessary (I)
Maintain a patent airway (I)
Evaluate the patient's breathing pattern for shortness of breath or diaphoresis (I)

Nutrition

Assist the patient with eating (I)
Incorporate the patient's food preferences into his or her diet (I)
Consult with the dietitian (I)

Communication

Support the patient through the frustration of speech change (I)
Encourage the patient to strive toward realistic goals (I)
Encourage patient acceptance of self-limitations (I)
Explore with the patient the reasons for self-criticism (I)
Encourage the patient when he or she attempts to speak (I)
Provide alternative means of communication (I)
Provide support for the patient's family (I)
Inform the patient as to what is expected of him or her in critical care (I)
Arrange situations that encourage the patient's autonomy (I)

Activity

Evaluate for abnormal physical activity or movement (I)
Encourage alternative rest and moderate activity periods (I)
Provide diversional activities (I)

Pain

> Discuss possible pain-relieving measures (I)
> Reduce physical discomfort that could interfere with cognitive functions (I)
> Prepare the patient for a painful experience (I)

Bibliography

Hickey, J. *Clinical practice of neurological and neurosurgical nursing.* Philadelphia: Lippincott, 1981.

Johanson, B., Dungca, C., Hoffmeister, D. & Wells, S. *Standards for critical care.* St. Louis: C. V. Mosby, 1985.

Roberts, S. *Physiological concepts and the critically ill patient.* Englewood Cliffs, N.J.: Prentice-Hall, 1985, pp. 448–498.

Wyngaarden, J. & Smith, L. *Cecil's textbook of medicine* (17th ed.). Philadelphia: W. B. Saunders, 1985.

Self-Care Deficit

DEFINITION

A self-care deficit occurs when an individual experiences impaired or cognitive functions, causing dependence upon others for one's physical needs.

ETIOLOGY

> Arthritis
> Multiple sclerosis
> Diabetes mellitus
> Hypothyroidism
> Parkinsonism
> Myasthenia gravis
> Lack of coordination
> Muscular weakness
> Paralysis
> CVA
> Cataracts
> Fractures
> Edema
> Glaucoma
> Contractures
> Immobility

Hemodynamic instrumentation
Trauma
Supportive devices
Invasive tubes
Casts
Pain
Depression
Anxiety

DEFINING CHARACTERISTICS

Regulatory Behaviors
Limited ability to ambulate
Weakness

Cognitive Behaviors
Inability to bathe, feed, dress, or toilet self
Limited ability to perform diabetic care

NURSING RESPONSIBILITIES

Assessment
Assess regulatory behaviors indicative of self-care deficit (I)
Assess cognitive behaviors indicative of self-care deficit (I)

Interventions

Fluid
Assist the patient with his or her toilet needs: bedpan, commode, or bathroom (I)

Aeration
Reduce meaningless stimuli (I)
Create an environment that encourages the patient to participate in self-care (I)

Nutrition
Assist the patient with his or her feeding needs (I)
Encourage the intake of foods enjoyed by the patient (I)

Communication
Listen to the patient's concerns, fears, and anxieties (I)
Allow the patient to ventilate his or her feelings and frustrations (I)

Provide knowledge as to ways in which the patient can participate in self-care (I)

Encourage patient self-performance (I)

Encourage patient acceptance of self-limitations (I)

Explore with the patient previous achievements or successes (I)

Encourage decision making (I)

Arrange situations that encourage the patient's autonomy (I)

Provide measures to increase the patient's self-confidence (I)

Reward the patient, both verbally and nonverbally, for self-care accomplishments (I)

Encourage family and friends to reward the patient verbally and nonverbally for self-care accomplishments (I)

Activity

Gradually increase the patient's responsibilities regarding activities of daily living (ADLs) (ID)

Change the patient's position q2h (I)

Develop an individualized teaching program for both patient and family (I)

Space the practice of self-care activities (I)

Encourage and reassure the patient that he or she can do ADLs provided that he or she takes frequent rest periods (I)

Assist the patient with ADLs while allowing him or her to do everything that he or she is able to do (I)

Pain

Administer prescribed analgesics (D)

Discuss possible pain-relieving measures (I)

Prepare the patient for a painful experience (I)

Bibliography

Carpenito, L. J. *Handbook of nursing diagnosis.* Philadelphia: Lippincott, 1984.

Gettrust, K., Ryan, S., & Engleman, D. *Applied nursing diagnosis.* New York: Wiley, 1985.

Kelly, M. *Nursing diagnosis source book.* Norwalk, Conn.: Appleton-Century-Crofts, 1985.

Kim, M. J., McFarland, G., & McLane, A. *Nursing diagnosis.* St. Louis: C. V. Mosby, 1984.

INJURY, POTENTIAL FOR
Potential for Injury, Facial Trauma

DEFINITION
A state in which the individual sustains traumatic injuries to the face.

ETIOLOGY
Facial lacerations
Facial fractures
    Nasal fracture
    Maxillary fracture
    Oribital blow-out fracture
    Zygomatic fracture
    Mandibular fracture

DEFINING CHARACTERISTICS
Regulatory Behaviors
Bleeding
Skin penetration
Palpable infraorbital rim fracture
Swelling
Limited eye movement in upward gaze
Pain
Bone or fragment displacement
Palpation of fracture
Trismus
Periorbital hematoma
Periorbital edema
Subconjunctival hemorrhage
Enophthalmos

Cognitive Behaviors
Anxiety
Restlessness
Agitation
Fear

NURSING RESPONSIBILITIES

Assessment

Assess regulatory behaviors indicative of facial trauma (I)

Assess the eyes for loss of vision, diplopia, foreign bodies, penetrating bodies, and hemorrhage (I)

Assess the face for malocclusion of teeth, tenderness to the touch, asymmetry of the infraorbital rim, zygomatic arch, anterior wall of the antrum, angles of the jaw, and lower borders of the mandible (I)

Assess the cerebrospinal fluid leaking from the nose or face (I)

Assess the patient's neurological status: pupillary changes, sensory/motor changes, vital signs, and level of consciousness (I)

Palpate peripheral pulses for quality and bilateral equality (I)

Auscultate the heart for rate, rhythm, and regularity (I)

Inspect for edema (I)

Auscultate the chest for abnormal breath sounds (I)

Auscultate the chest for respiratory rate, rhythm, and regularity (I)

Interventions

Fluid

Administer prescribed IV fluid (D)

Administer prescribed medications (D)

Measure arterial blood pressure and MAP (I)

Measure intake and output (I)

Apply direct pressure to a bleeding site when possible (I)

Evaluate laboratory studies (I)

Aeration

Insert a nasopharyngeal airway, especially when edema is present (D)

Administer oxygen at the prescribed percentage and flow rate (D)

Maintain a patent airway (I)

Clear any airway obstruction (I)

Evaluate adequacy of breathing pattern (I)

Evaluate the breathing pattern for shortness of breath or dyspnea (I)

Evaluate arterial blood gasses (I)

Nutrition
NPO

Insert nasogastric tube or oral gastric tube if possible (ID)

Communication
Provide knowledge regarding the extent of the injury and treatment modalities (ID)

Provide the family with knowledge regarding the patient's injuries (ID)

Reduce the patient's anxiety level (I)

Activity
Immobilize the patient until the possibility of cervical injury can be ruled out (I)

Reduce meaningless environmental stimuli (I)

Pain
Administer prescribed analgesics (D)

Evaluate the type, location, and duration of pain (I)

Bibliography

Budassi, S. & Barber, J. *Mosby's manual of emergency care practices and procedures* (2nd ed.). St. Louis: C. V. Mosby, 1984.

Sheehy, S. & Barber, J. *Emergency nursing principles and practice.* St. Louis: C. V. Mosby, 1985.

Injury, Limb Trauma

DEFINITION
Injury to the soft tissue, peripheral nerves, fractures, or traumatic amputation constitutes limb trauma.

ETIOLOGY
Soft tissue injuries
    Abrasion
    Avulsion
    Contusion
    Laceration

Puncture
Abscess
Hematoma
Gunshot wound
Impaling injury
Crush injury
Knee injury
Strains
Sprains
Peripheral nerve injuries
Fractures
    Clavicular
    Shoulder
    Scapular
    Humeral shaft
    Elbow
    Radius or ulna
    Wrist
    Hand
    Finger
    Pelvis
    Hip
    Femoral
    Knee
    Patellar
    Tibia
    Fibula
    Ankle
    Foot
    Heel
    Toes
Dislocation
    Acromioclavicular separation
    Shoulder
    Elbow
    Wrist
    Hand or finger
    Hip
    Knee
    Patella

Ankle
Traumatic amputations

DEFINING CHARACTERISTICS

Regulatory Behaviors

Swelling
Ecchymosis
Pain
  Local
  Sharp
Tenderness
  Joint(s)
  Sacroiliac
Spasm
Inability to use limb for a short period of time
Deformity
Positive Thompson's sign
Crepitus
Decreased circulation to the hand
Paresis
Hemiparesis
External rotation of the hip and leg
Inability to bear weight
Shortening of the limb
Discoloration

Cognitive Behaviors

Anger
Anxiety
Fear
Apprehension

NURSING RESPONSIBILITIES

Assessment

Assess regulatory behaviors indicative of limb injury (I)
Assess other major trauma sites: head, cervical, spine, chest, and abdomen (I)
Observe the side or therapeutic effects of prescribed medications (I)
Auscultate the chest for respiratory rate, rhythm, and regularity (I)

Interventions

Fluid

Administer prescribed IV fluids (D)

Administer prescribed medications (D)

Administer a blood transfusion if necessary (D)

Irrigate the wound site with normal saline (ID)

Apply a dry, sterile dressing over the wound (ID)

Apply a slight compression dressing (ID)

Regulate the IV flow rate and check for patency (I)

Evaluate the vascular status of the limb before and after immobilization: pulses distal to the trauma, color, temperature, and capillary refill (I)

Measure blood pressure (I)

Evaluate the amount of blood loss (I)

Measure intake and output (I)

Evaluate the neurological status of the limb before and after immobilization (I)

Evaluate the skin for color and lacerations (I)

Evaluate the hemoglobin and hematrocrit studies (I)

Evaluate the extremities for swelling, discoloration, contusions, abrasions, or obvious deformities (I)

Apply a cold pack to the area (I)

Aeration

Administer humidified oxygen at the prescribed flow rate (D)

Reduce extraneous stimuli in the environment (I)

Nutrition

NPO

Communication

Provide knowledge regarding the injury and treatment (ID)

Reduce the patient's anxiety level (I)

Listen to the patient's concerns regarding the possible loss of his or her limb (I)

Activity

Immobilize the traumatized limb both above and below the trauma site (ID)

Splint the limb (ID)

    Elevate the limb if possible (I)
    Protect the patient's head and cervical spine (I)

Pain

    Administer the prescribed analgesics (D)
    Evaluate the extent of the patient's limb pain (I)

Bibliography

Budassi, S. & Barber, J. *Mosby's manual of emergency care practices and procedures.* St. Louis: C. V. Mosby, 1984.
Sheehy, S. & Barber, J. *Emergency nursing principles and practice* (2nd ed.). St. Louis: C. V. Mosby, 1985.

Potential for Injury, Spinal Cord Trauma

DEFINITION

A state in which the individual experiences spinal cord trauma, causing a disruption of messages between the brain and the body in the form of electrical inputs through sensory/motor tracts.

ETIOLOGY

    Extension/hyperflexion injury
    Spinal shock
    Lesions of
        $C_3–C_7$
        $T_1–T_2$
        T_7
        L_4

DEFINING CHARACTERISTICS

Regulatory Behaviors

    Neck tenderness and pain
    Weakness in the extremities
    Numbness and tingling
    Decreased motor activity distal to the injury
    Decreased anal sphincter tone
    Pain on careful palpation of the spine
    Decreased blood pressure in spinal shock
    Priapism

Cognitive Behaviors
  Anxiety
  Fear
  Pain
  Hopelessness
  Powerlessness
  Depression
  Apprehension

NURSING RESPONSIBILITIES

Assessment

  Assess regulatory behaviors indicative of spinal cord trauma
    (I)
  Assess the exact cause of the injury (I)
  Monitor the ECG pattern continuously (I)
  Auscultate the chest for adventitious breath sounds (I)

Interventions

Fluid

  Administer prescribed IV fluids (D)
  Administer prescribed medications (D)
  Evaluate laboratory studies (I)
  Measure blood pressure and MAP (I)
  Evaluate the skin for color, temperature, and diaphoresis (I)

Aeration

  Provide oxygen at the prescribed percentage and flow rate
    (D)
  Maintain a patent airway (I)
  Suction the patient as necessary (I)
  Measure intake and output (I)
  Evaluate the patient's ability to utilize respiratory muscles
    (I)

Nutrition

  Assist the patient with eating (I)
  Incorporate the patient's preferences into his or her diet (I)
  Insert a nasogastric tube (I)
  Measure the patient's nasogastric output (I)

Communication

Reduce the patient's anxiety level (I)

Listen to the patient's concerns (I)

Support the family throughout the patient's hospitalization (I)

Activity

Evaluate the patient for touch sensation (I)

Evaluate the patient for paresthesia or paralysis (I)

Evaluate the patient's ability to grip with the hands (I)

Evaluate the patient's ability to wiggle his or her toes (I)

Immobilize the neck (I)

Pain

Administer prescribed medications (D)

Evaluate the type, location, and duration of pain (I)

Bibliography

Budassi, S. & Barber, J. *Mosby's manual of emergency care practices and procedures.* St. Louis: C. V. Mosby, 1984.

Sheehy, S. & Barber, J. *Emergency nursing principles and practice* (2nd ed.). St. Louis: C. V. Mosby, 1985.

GENITOURINARY/RENAL SYSTEM

In assessing the critically ill patient's renal status, the nurse applies his or her knowledge of the genitourinary/renal system. The nurse incorporates this knowledge, including data collected from physical assessment, into formulating a collaborative nursing diagnosis for these systems.

FLUID-VOLUME DEFICIT

Intracellular-Extracellular Fluid-Volume Deficit, Dehydration

DEFINITION

Dehydration is the loss of water from the extracellular fluid compartment, causing some of the intracellular water to pass into the extracellular compartments by osmosis, resulting in an increase in the concentration of extracellular–intracellular solute.

ETIOLOGY
Fever
    Reduced fluid intake
        Comatose patient
        Esophageal obstruction
        Pyloric obstruction
    Diabetic insipidus
    Nephrogenic diabetic insipidus
    Diabetes mellitus
    Hypokalemia
    Hypercalcemia
    Correction of obstruction uropathy
    Intensive diuretic therapy
    Drugs
        Demeclocycline
        Amphotericin B
    Renal disease
        Addison's disease
        Hyporeninemic hypoaldosteronism
        Interstitial nephritis
        Renal tubular acidosis
        Bartier's syndrome
        Osmotic diuresis
        Chronic renal failure
    Sweating
    Burns
    Vomiting
    Diarrhea
    Tube drainage
    Gastrointestinal fistula

DEFINING CHARACTERISTICS

Regulatory Behaviors
    Flushed skin
    Acute weight loss
    Dry mucous membrane
    Weakness

Cold extremities
Oliguria
Tachycardia
Hypotension
Hyperpnea
Decreased CVP
Decreased PCWP
Diaphoresis
Fatigue
Thirst
Decreased skin turgor

Cognitive Behaviors
Hallucination
Delirium
Change in the level of consciousness
Giddiness
Dizziness
Restlessness

NURSING RESPONSIBILITIES

Assessment
Assess regulatory behaviors indicative of dehydration (I)
Assess cognitive behaviors indicative of dehydration (I)
Monitor the ECG pattern continuously (I)
Auscultate the chest for abnormal heart sounds (I)
Inspect the jugular veins (I)
Palpate for the presence of peripheral pulses and check for bilateral equality (I)
Inspect skin turgor and mucous membranes for hydration status (I)
Auscultate the chest for respiratory rate, rhythm, and regularity (I)
Inspect chest movement for labored breathing and symmetry (I)

Interventions

Fluid
Administer appropriate IV fluids (D)
2.5 to 5% dextrose/water (D/W)
Sodium replacement

Increase fluid intake to 2000 to 3000 ml/day (1500 ml/m^2 of body surface (D)

Measure blood pressure and MAP (I)

Measure intake, urine volume, and specific gravity (I)

Regulate the IV flow rate and check for patency (I)

Measure the output from nasogastric tubes, rectal tubes, and/or diarrhea, etc. (I)

Evaluate data from hemodynamic parameters: PAP, PCWP, CVP, and CO (I)

Evaluate hematocrit, hemoglobin, serum electrolytes, creatinine, and BUN (I)

Aeration

Evaluate the skin for color, temperature, and moisture (I)

Provide humidified oxygen via mask, nasal catheter, or nasal prongs at the prescribed percentage and flow rate (I)

Evaluate arterial blood gasses (I)

Encourage the patient to deep-breathe (I)

Nutrition

Provide assistance for the patient unable to eat or drink independently (I)

Encourage the patient to maintain the prescribed diet (I)

Provide cold or warm fluid, depending upon the patient's preference (I)

Communication

Inform the physician of any changes in the patient's condition (I)

Provide knowledge regarding diagnostic procedures or supportive devices (I)

Reduce the patient's anxiety level (I)

Activity

Change the patient's position q2h (I)

Provide alternate periods of rest and moderate activity (I)

Encourage the use of passive and active range-of-motion exercises (I)

Pain

Administer analgesics as prescribed (D)

Evaluate the type, location, and duration of pain (I)

Reassure the patient that any pain will subside or be relieved (I)

Discuss possible pain-relieving measures (I)

Bibliography

Gettrust, K. Ryan, S., & Engleman, D. *Applied nursing diagnosis.* New
York: Wiley, 1985.

Kim, M. J., McFarland, G., & McLane, A. *Nursing diagnosis.* St. Louis:
C. V. Mosby, 1984.

Wyngaarden, J. & Smith, L. *Cecil textbook of medicine.* Philadelphia:
W. B. Saunders, 1985.

Intracellular Electrolyte Deficit, Hypokalemia

DEFINITION

Mild hypokalemia is defined as a level between 3.0 and 3.4
mEq/L and severe hypokalemia is a level below 3.0 mEq/L.

ETIOLOGY

Inadequate intake

Excess renal loss

    Mineralocorticoid excess

    Barlter's syndrome

    Diuresis

    Chronic metabolic alkalosis

    Antibiotics

        Carbenicillin

        Gentamicin

        Amphotercin B

    Renal tubular acidosis

    Liddle's syndrome

    Acute leukemia

    Ureterosigmoidostomy

Gastrointestinal losses

    Vomiting

    Diarrhea

    Villous adenoma

Extracellular fluid–intracellular fluid shifts

    Acute alkalosis

    Hypokalemic periodic paralysis

Barium ingestion
Insulin therapy
Vitamin B_{12} therapy

DEFINING CHARACTERISTICS

Regulatory Behaviors
Muscular weakness
Areflexic paralysis
Paralytic ileus
Impaired ventilation
Arrhythmias
Anorexia
Nausea
Vomiting
Hypotension
Enhanced digitalis effect

Cognitive Behaviors
Lassitude
Expression of discomfort
Uneasy feeling
Drowsiness
Coma

NURSING RESPONSIBILITIES

Assessment
Assess regulatory behaviors indicative of hypokalemia (I)
Assess cognitive behaviors indicative of hypokalemia (I)
Assess the patient's neurological status (I)
Monitor the ECG pattern continuously (I)
Observe the side or therapeutic effects of prescribed medications (I)
Monitor the ECG for signs of digitalis toxicity (I)
Auscultate the heart for rate, rhythm, and regularity (I)
Auscultate the chest for adventitious breath sounds (I)
Auscultate the chest for respiratory rate, rhythm, and regularity (I)

Interventions

Fluid
Replace lost potassium with oral supplements and IV potassium chloride (D)

Evaluate serum electrolyte levels (I)

Measure the components of ECG reflecting hypokalemia (I)
    Decreased amplitude and broadening of T waves
    Prominent U waves
    Sagging ST segments
    Atrioventricular block
    Cardiac arrest

Evaluate arterial blood gasses (I)

Measure urinary volume and specific gravity (I)

Estimate the degree of potassium lost in drainage (gastric aspirate and diarrhea) to aid in calculating the patient's total body potassium balance (I)

Regulate IV replacement of potassium chloride—slowly, so as to prevent hyperkalemia and ventricular arrhythmias (I)

Evaluate the skin for color, temperature, and presence of diaphoresis (I)

Aeration

Provide oxygen at the prescribed percentage and flow rate (D)

Provide ventilatory support as needed (D)

Evaluate arterial blood gasses (I)

Reduce extraneous environmental stimuli (I)

Nutrition

Provide a diet rich in potassium (ID)
    Natural fruits: oranges, bananas, peaches, strawberries, and tomatoes
    Juices
    Dried fruits: apricots, dates, and raisins

Consult with the dietitian (I)

Assist the patient with his or her diet (I)

Communication

Reduce the patient's anxiety level (I)

Listen to the patient's concerns and fears (I)

Provide knowledge regarding the causes of hypokalemia (I)

Activity

Estimate the degree of muscular weakness (I)

Provide rest periods between nursing interventions (I)

Encourage moderate activity or ambulation with supervision (I)

Pain

Administer analgesics as prescribed (D)
Evaluate the type, location, and duration of pain (I)
Reassure the patient that the pain will subside (I)

Bibliography

Borg, N., Nikas, D., Stark, J., & Williams, S. *Core curriculum critical care nursing.* Philadelphia: W. B. Saunders, 1981.

Krupp, M., Chatton, M., & Werdeger, D. *Current medical diagnosis and treatment.* Los Altos, Calif.: Lange Medical Publications, 1985.

Wyngaarden, J. & Smith, L. *Cecil textbook of medicine* (17th ed.). Philadelphia: W. B. Saunders, 1985.

Extracellular Electrolyte Deficit, Hyponatremia

DEFINITION

Hyponatremia is present when the sodium level is less than
138 mEq/L.

ETIOLOGY

Diuretic excess
Mineralocorticoid deficiency
Salt-losing nephritis
Renal tubular acidosis with bicarbonaturia
Vomiting
Diarrhea
Third-space burns
Pancreatitis
Traumatized muscle
Glucocorticoid deficiency
Hypothyroidism
Pain
Emotion
Drugs
Syndrome of inappropriate antidiuretic hormone (ADH)
secretion
Nephrotic syndrome
Cirrhosis

Cardiac failure
Chronic renal failure

DEFINING CHARACTERISTICS

Regulatory Behaviors
Headache
Seizures
Weakness
Coma
Death

Cognitive Behaviors
Lethargy
Obtundation
Somnolence

NURSING RESPONSIBILITIES

Assessment
Assess regulatory behaviors indicative of hyponatremia (I)
Assess cognitive behaviors indicative of hyponatremia (I)
Monitor the ECG pattern continuously (I)
Assess the patient's neurological status (I)
Auscultate the heart for rate, rhythm, and regularity (I)
Palpate for the presence of peripheral pulses and check for bilateral equality (I)
Inspect skin turgor for evidence of dehydration (I)
Auscultate the chest for abnormal breath sounds (I)
Auscultate the chest for adventitious breath sounds (I)
Inspect chest movement for labored breathing and symmetry (I)

Intervention

Fluid
Administer prescribed IV fluids (D)
Isotonic saline
3 to 5% saline
Replace electrolytes (D)
Measure blood pressure and MAP (I)
Evaluate serum electrolytes (I)
Measure intake, output, and specific gravity (I)
Regulate the IV flow rate and check for patency (I)

Aeration

Provide oxygen at the prescribed percentage and flow rate (D)

Evaluate arterial blood gasses (I)

Nutrition

Encourage the patient to maintain the prescribed diet (I)

Assist the patient with eating if necessary (I)

Communication

Provide knowledge regarding diagnostic procedures and supportive devices (I)

Listen to the patient's concerns (I)

Inform the physician of any changes in the patient's condition (I)

Activity

Change the patient's position q2h (I)

Evaluate any alteration in the patient's thought process (I)

Provide diversional activities (I)

Provide alternate periods of rest and moderate activity (I)

Pain

Administer analgesics as prescribed (D)

Evaluate the type, location, and duration of pain (I)

Bibliography

Borg, N., Nikas, D., Stark, J., & Williams, S. *Core curriculum for critical care nursing.* Philadelphia: W. B. Saunders, 1981.

Roberts, S. *Physiological concepts and the critically ill patient.* Englewood Cliffs, N.J.: Prentice-Hall, 1985, pp. 340-385.

Wyngaarden, J. & Smith, L. *Cecil textbook of medicine* (17th ed.). Philadelphia: W. B. Saunders, 1985.

Intracellular Electrolyte Deficit, Hypomagnesium

DEFINITION

Hypomagnesium is defined as a serum magnesium level less than 1.5 mEq/L.

ETIOLOGY

Diminished absorption or intake

Malabsorption

Chronic diarrhea
Laxative abuse
Prolonged gastrointestinal suction
Small bowel bypass
Malnutrition
Alcoholism
Parenteral alimentation with inadequate magnesium con-
tent
Increased loss
Diabetic ketoacidosis
Diuretic therapy
Diarrhea
Hyperaldosteronism
Barlter's syndrome
Hypercalcuria
Renal magnesium wasting
Unexplained
Hyperparathyroidism
Postparathyroidectomy
Vitamin D therapy
Induced by aminoglycoside antibiotics, cisplatin

DEFINING CHARACTERISTICS

Regulatory Behaviors
Atheloid movements
Jerking
Coarse and flapping tremors
Positive Babinski response
Nystagmus
Tachycardia
Ventricular arrhythmias

Cognitive Behaviors
Irritability
Confusion
Disorientation
Restlessness

NURSING RESPONSIBILITIES

Assessment
Assess regulatory behaviors indicative of hypomagnesium (I)

Assess cognitive behaviors indicative of hypomagnesium (I)
Monitor the ECG pattern continuously (I)
Assess the patient's neurological status (I)
Observe the side or therapeutic effects of prescribed medi-
cations (I)
Auscultate the chest for respiratory rate, rhythm, and regu-
larity (I)

Interventions

Fluid

Administer prescribed medications (D)
  Magnesium sulfate
    8.33 mmol/day intramuscularly in 4 divided doses
  Magnesium oxide
    250 to 500 mg 2-4 times daily
Administer IV fluids as prescribed (D)
  Magnesium chloride or sulfate
    5-30 mmol/day during the period of severe deficit,
    followed by 5 mmol/day for maintenance
Evaluate serum magnesium levels (I)
Measure blood pressure and MAP (I)
Measure intake and output (I)
Measure the amount of drainage from nasogastric suction (I)

Aeration

Evaluate the breathing pattern for shortness of breath or
dyspnea (I)
Reduce meaningless environmental stimuli (I)

Nutrition

Provide a diet adequate to meet the nutritional needs of the
patient, thereby avoiding malnutrition (I)
Consult with the dietitian (I)

Communication

Inform the physician of any significant changes in serum
electrolytes, including magnesium (I)
Provide knowledge regarding the causes of hypomagnesium
(I)
Instruct the patient regarding the relationship between
alcoholism, malnutrition, and hypomagnesium (I)
Listen to the patient's concerns regarding the critical envi-
ronment (I)

Activity
   Provide diversional activities (I)
   Evaluate any alterations in the patient's thought process (I)
   Encourage physical mobility (I)

Pain
   Administer prescribed medications (D)
   Evaluate the presence of pain (I)

Bibliography

Borg, N., Nikas, D., Stark, J., & Williams. S. *Core curriculum for critical care nursing.* Philadelphia: W. B. Saunders, 1981.

Krupp, M., Chalton, M., & Werdegar, D. *Current medical diagnosis and treatment.* Los Altos, Calif.: Lange Medical Publications, 1985.

Actual Whole Blood and Plasma Volume Deficit, Traumatic Shock

DEFINITION

Traumatic shock can occur from hemorrhage and from severe and/or extensive contusions to the body, causing sufficient damage to the capillaries to result in increased capillary permeability, with a subsequent escape of plasma from the vascular compartment into the interstitial compartment.

ETIOLOGY

   Multiple fractures and internal injuries from a fall
   Blunt penetrating wound
   Gunshot
   Automobile accident

DEFINING CHARACTERISTICS

Regulatory Behaviors
   Hypoxia
   Hypotension
   Tachycardia
   Weak pulse
   Convulsion
   Tachypnea
   Oliguria
   Pallor
   Cyanosis

Weakness
Fatigue

Cognitive Behaviors
Depression
Loss of consciousness
Restlessness
Hyperactivity
Apprehension
Delirium

NURSING RESPONSIBILITIES

Assessment

Inspect the patient to determine the site of injury (ID)
Assess regulatory behaviors indicative of traumatic shock (I)
Assess cognitive behaviors indicative of traumatic shock (I)
Monitor the ECG pattern continuously (I)
Observe the side or therapeutic effects of prescribed medications (I)
Assess the patient's neurological status (I)
Auscultate the chest for abnormal breath sounds (I)
Auscultate the chest for respiratory rate, rhythm, and regularity (I)
Inspect for bleeding (I)
Palpate peripheral pulses for quality and bilateral equality (I)
Palpate the chest for an abnormal precordial thrust (I)
Inspect the chest for precordial bulge (I)
Inspect the skin for pallor or cyanosis (I)
Auscultate the chest for respiratory rate, rhythm, and regularity (I)
Auscultate the chest for adventitious breath sounds (I)
Percuss the chest for abnormal resonance (I)
Inspect for evidence of abnormal body movement (I)
Inspect the abdomen for distension (I)
Palpate the abdomen for tenderness or rigidity (I)

Interventions

Fluid

Administer prescribed medications (D)
NaHCO₃
Insulin

Replace circulating blood volume through the use of plasma or plasma expanders (I)

Evaluate laboratory values (I)

Apply direct pressure to the local bleeding site (I)

Evaluate the patient's vital signs and neurological status (I)

Measure all output, including drainage, bleeding, and urinary volume (I)

Evaluate blood studies for abnormal clotting mechanisms (I)

Evaluate the skin for color, temperature, and presence of diaphoresis (I)

Aeration

Provide oxygen at the prescribed percentage and flow rate (D)

Maintain adequate ventilation through the use of continuous ventilatory support if necessary (ID)

Measure the amount of chest-tube drainage (I)

Evaluate the breathing pattern for shortness of breath or dyspnea (I)

Evaluate for airway obstruction (I)

Establish and maintain a patent airway (I)

Evaluate chest movement for labored breathing and symmetry (I)

Evaluate arterial blood gasses (I)

Nutrition

Insert nasogastric tube and connect to continuous or intermittent suction as temporarily prescribed (ID)

NPO

Communication

Inform the family of the patient's condition and progress (ID)

Reduce the patient's anxiety level during the initial stages of shock (I)

Inform the physician of changes in the patient's laboratory, diagnostic, or physiological status (I)

Support and reassure the patient through the traumatic shock experience (I)

Activity

Immobilize the patient until the extent of his or her injuries can be evaluated (I)

Evaluate any changes in sensory–motor status (I)

Evaluate any alterations in the patient's thought process (I)

Evaluate any alteration in the patient's level of consciousness (I)

Protect the patient if he or she experiences seizure activity (I)

Evaluate the eyes for pupil size, equality, and response to light (I)

Pain

Administer the prescribed medications (D)

Evaluate for the presence of pain (I)

Evaluate the type, location, and duration of pain (I)

Bibliography

Bordicks, K. *Patterns of shock implications for nursing care* (2nd ed.). New York: Macmillan, 1980.

Borg, N., Nikas, D., Stark, J., & Williams, S. *Core curriculum for critical care nursing.* Philadelphia: W. B. Saunders, 1981.

Gettrust, K., Ryan, S., & Engleman, D. *Applied nursing diagnosis.* New York: Wiley, 1985.

FLUID VOLUME, EXCESS

Extracellular Fluid Volume, Excess, Edema

DEFINITION

Edema is the abnormal accumulation of extravascular interstitial fluid of a magnitude sufficient to be clinically detectable.

ETIOLOGY

Disturbed, startling forces

SVP increase

Right heart failure

Constrictive pericarditis

Local venous pressure increases

Left heart failure

Vena cava obstruction

Reduced oncotic pressure

Nephrotic syndrome

Combined disorders

Cirrhosis

Primary hormone excess
    Primary aldosteronism
    Cushing's syndrome
Primary renal sodium retention
    Acute glomerulonephritis

DEFINING CHARACTERISTICS

Regulatory Behaviors
Weight gain
Anasarca
Orthopnea
Crackles
S_3
Decreased hemoglobin
Decreased hematocrit
Hypertension
Jugular-vein distension
Increased PAP
Increased PCWP
Oliguria
Azotemia

Cognitive Behaviors
Changes in mental status
Restlessness
Anxiety
Apprehension

NURSING RESPONSIBILITIES

Assessment
Assess regulatory behaviors indicative of edema (I)
Assess cognitive behaviors indicative of edema (I)
Monitor the ECG pattern continuously (I)
Observe the side or therapeutic effects of prescribed medications (I)
Assess the patient's neurological status (I)
Auscultate the chest for abnormal heart sounds: S_3 (I)
Inspect the jugular veins (I)
Palpate for the presence of peripheral pulses and check for bilateral equality (I)

Auscultate the chest for rales (I)
Auscultate the chest for respiratory rate, rhythm, and regularity (I)

Interventions

Fluid

Administer prescribed diuretics (D)
    Proximal diuretics
        Acetazolamide
        Metolazone
    Loop diuretics
        Furosemide
        Ethacrynic acid
    Early distal diuretics
        Thiazide
        Metolazone
    Late distal diuretics
        Aldosterone antagonists
            Spironolactone
        Nonaldosterone antagonists
            Triamterene
Measure arterial blood pressure and MAP (I)
Evaluate data from hemodynamic parameters: CVP, PAP, PCWP, and CO (I)
Measure urinary volume and specific gravity q1h (I)
Measure and restrict oral and IV fluid intake (I)
Measure nasogastric tube drainage (I)
Evaluate the patient's weight (I)
Regulate the IV flow rate and check for patency (I)
Evaluate the skin for the presence of edema (I)
Evaluate hemoglobin, hematocrit, serum electrolytes, BUN, and creatinine (I)

Aeration

Provide humidified oxygen via mask, nasal catheter, or nasal prongs at the prescribed percentage and flow rate (D)
Provide ventilatory support (D)
Evaluate the chest for vocal and tactile fremitus (I)
Suction the patient via mouth, endotracheal tube, or tracheostomy while using strict aseptic techniques (I)

Encourage the patient to cough, turn, and deep-breathe (I)

Evaluate arterial blood gasses (I)

Inspect chest movement for labored breathing and symmetry (I)

Nutrition

Provide the patient with a low-salt diet (D)

Encourage the patient to eat the prescribed diet (I)

Restrict fluid intake (I)

Communication

Provide knowledge regarding diagnostic procedures or supportive devices (I)

Reduce the patient's anxiety level (I)

Inform the physician of any changes in the patient's condition (I)

Listen to the patient's concerns, fears, and anxieties (I)

Support the family throughout the patient's hospitalization (I)

Activity

Change the patient's position q2h (I)

Elevate the head of the bed (I)

Elevate the edematous body part (I)

Provide periods of rest and moderate activity (I)

Apply antiembolic or support stockings (I)

Encourage the use of diversional activities (I)

Pain

Administer analgesics as prescribed (D)

Evaluate the type, location, and duration of pain (I)

Bibliography

Kim, M. J., McFarland, G., & McLane, A. *Nursing diagnosis.* St. Louis: C. V. Mosby, 1984.

Wyngaarden, J. & Smith, L. *Cecil textbook of medicine* (17th ed.). Philadelphia: W. B. Saunders, 1985.

Intracellular Electrolyte Excess, Hyperkalemia

DEFINITION

Hyperkalemia is defined as a serum potassium level of greater than 5.0 mEq/L or a plasma potassium level of greater than 4.5 mEq/L.

ETIOLOGY
Diminished renal excretion
    Reduced glomerular filtration rate (GFR)
        Acute oliguric renal failure
        Chronic renal failure
    Reduced tubular secretion
        Addison's disease
        Hyporeninemic hypoaldosteronism
        Potassium-sparing diuretics
Transcellular shifts
    Acidosis
    Cell destruction
    Trauma
    Burns
    Rhabdomolysis
    Hemolysis
    Tumorlysis
Hyperkalemic periodic paralysis
Diabetic hyperglycemia
    Insulin dependence plus aldosterone lack
Depolarizing muscle paralysis
    Succinylcholine

NURSING CHARACTERISTICS

Regulatory Behaviors
Muscle weakness
Paralysis of respiratory muscles
Fatigue
Asystole
Abdominal distension
Diarrhea
Oliguria

Cognitive Behaviors
Anxiety
Apprehension
Expression of discomfort
Tiredness
Apathy
Confusion

NURSING RESPONSIBILITIES

Assessment

Assess regulatory behaviors indicative of hyperkalemia (I)
Assess cognitive behaviors indicative of hyperkalemia (I)
Observe the side or therapeutic effects of prescribed drugs (I)
Auscultate the heart for rate, rhythm, and regularity (I)
Auscultate the heart for abnormal heart sounds (I)
Auscultate the chest for adventitious breath sounds (I)
Percuss the posterior chest for decreased diaphragmatic descent (I)
Auscultate the abdomen for abnormal bowel sounds (I)
Inspect the abdomen for distension (I)
Inspect the abdomen for vein engorgement (I)

Interventions

Fluid

Administer prescribed medications (D)
 Calcium gluconate 10%
  10–20 mL in 2–3 min; may repeat×1
 Sodium bicarbonate (NaHCO₃)
  1 ampule in 5 min; may repeat in 1 min
 50% glucose
  1 ampule in 5 min; follow with a 10% glucose infusion
 Regular insulin
  10–20 units/100 g glucose
 Kayexalate
  20–50 gm in 100–200 ml of 20% sorbitol
 Thiazide diuretics
Evaluate the components of the ECG reflecting hyperkalemia (I)
 Peaked T waves of increased amplitude
 Atrial arrest
 Spread in QRS
 Biphasic QRS–T complexes
 Ventricular fibrillation
 Cardiac arrest
Evaluate serum electrolytes (I)
Measure urinary output and diarrhea output (I)
Measure intake (I)

Aeration

Evaluate the respiratory rate and rhythm for evidence of respiratory muscle paralysis (I)

Establish and maintain a patent airway (I)

Evaluate the skin for cyanosis (I)

Evaluate the breathing pattern for shortness of breath or dyspnea (I)

Nutrition

Eliminate foods high in potassium until the patient's condition stabilizes (I)

Assist the patient with eating (I)

Communication

Listen to the patient's concerns (I)

Reduce the patient's anxiety level (I)

Support the patient through difficult diagnostic procedures or treatment interventions (I)

Activity

Provide adequate rest periods for the fatigued patient (I)

Apply appropriate antiseptic around the IV tubing connections to prevent infection (I)

Change the patient's position q2h (I)

Pain

Administer analgesics as prescribed (D)

Reduce physical discomfort that could interfere with the patient's cognitive function (I)

Evaluate the type, location, and duration of pain (I)

Bibliography

Borg, N., Nikas, D., Stark, J., & Williams. S. *Core curriculum for critical care nursing.* Philadelphia: W. B. Saunders, 1981.

Krupp, M., Chatton, M., & Werdegar, D. *Current medical diagnosis and treatment.* Los Altos, Calif.: Lange Medical Publications, 1985.

Wyngaarden, J. & Smith, L. *Cecil textbook of medicine* (17th ed.). Philadelphia: W. B. Saunders, 1985.

Extracellular Electrolyte Excess, Hypernatremia

DEFINITION

Hypernatremia is present when the sodium is greater than 144 meq/L.

ETIOLOGY
    Impaired thirst
        Coma
        Essential hypernatremia
    Solute diuresis
        Osmotic diuresis
            Diabetic ketoacidosis
            Nonketotic hyperosmolar coma
            Mannitol administration
    Excessive water losses
        Renal
            Pituitary diabetes insipidus
        Extrarenal
            Sweating
    Other
        Primary hyperaldosteronism
        Cushing's syndrome
        Sodium chloride tablets

DEFINING CHARACTERISTICS

Regulatory Behaviors
    Twitching
    Muscle weakness
    Seizure
    Coma
    Death
    Respiratory paralysis

Cognitive Behaviors
    Lethargy
    Altered mental status
    Difficulty concentrating

NURSING RESPONSIBILITIES

Assessment
    Assess regulatory behaviors indicative of hypernatremia (I)
    Assess cognitive behaviors indicative of hypernatremia (I)
    Monitor the ECG pattern continuously (I)
    Assess the patient's neurological status (I)
    Auscultate the heart for rate, rhythm, and regularity (I)

Inspect the jugular veins for distension (I)
Inspect for edema (I)
Auscultate the chest for adventitious breath sounds (I)
Inspect for cyanosis (I)
Auscultate the chest for respiratory rate, rhythm, and regularity (I)

Interventions

Fluid

Administer prescribed medications (D)
Administer IV fluids as prescribed (D)
  5% D/W
  2.5% D/¼ normal saline (N/S)
Measure blood pressure and MAP (I)
Measure intake, output, and specific gravity (I)
Evaluate the skin for color, temperature, and presence of diaphoresis (I)
Evaluate laboratory studies (I)

Aeration

Provide oxygen at the prescribed percentage and flow rate (D)
Evaluate arterial blood gasses (I)
Evaluate the breathing pattern for shortness of breath or dyspnea (I)
Reduce meaningless environmental stimuli (I)
Maintain a patent airway (I)

Nutrition

Encourage the patient to eat the prescribed diet (I)
Assist the patient with eating (I)

Communication

Provide knowledge regarding the causes of hypernatremia (I)
Reduce the patient's anxiety level (I)
Provide a spiritual support system if desired (I)
Listen to the family's concerns (I)

Activity

Reduce physical activity until the patient no longer experiences muscle weakness (I)
Prevent injuries during seizure activity (I)

Evaluate any alteration in the patient's thought process (I)
Provide diversional activity (I)

Pain
Evaluate for the presence of pain (I)
Evaluate the type, location, and duration of pain (I)
Administer prescribed medications (I)

Bibliography

Borg, N., Nikas, D., Stark, J., & Williams, S. *Core curriculum for critical care nursing.* Philadelphia: W. B. Saunders, 1981.

Roberts, S. *Physiological concepts and the critically ill patient.* Englewood Cliffs, N.J.: Prentice-Hall, 1985, pp. 340–385.

Wyngaarden, J. & Smith, L. *Cecil textbook of medicine* (17th ed.). Philadelphia: W. B. Saunders, 1985.

Intracellular Electrolyte Excess, Hypermagnesium

DEFINITION
Hypermagnesium is defined as a serum magnesium level greater than 2.5 mEq/L.

ETIOLOGY
Renal insufficiency
Magnesium sulfate as a cathartic
High doses of antacids

DEFINING CHARACTERISTICS

Regulatory Behaviors
Muscle weakness
Hypotension
Respiratory muscle paralysis
Death
Cardiac arrest
Asystole

Cognitive Behaviors
Sedation
Confusion

NURSING RESPONSIBILITIES

Assessment

Assess regulatory behaviors indicative of hypermagnesium (I)

Assess cognitive behaviors indicative of hypermagnesium (I)

Monitor the ECG pattern continuously (I)

Assess the patient's neurological status (I)

Auscultate the chest for respiratory rate, rhythm, and regularity (I)

Interventions

Fluid

Administer prescribed medications (D)

> Calcium acts as an antagonist to magnesium

Assist the physician with peritoneal dialysis (ID)

Measure the ECG components reflective of hypermagnesium (I)

> Increased P-R interval
> Broadened QRS complexes
> Elevated T waves

Regulate both the amount of fluid given and drainage via peritoneal dialysis (I)

Measure blood pressure and MAP (I)

Measure intake and output (I)

Evaluate serum electrolytes (I)

Evaluate the skin for color, temperature, and presence of diaphoresis (I)

Aeration

Provide oxygen via mask, nasal catheter, or nasal prongs at the prescribed percentage and flow rate (D)

Evaluate arterial blood gasses (I)

Reduce meaningless environmental stimuli (I)

Nutrition

Encourage the patient to eat the prescribed diet (I)

Incorporate the patient's food preferences into his or her diet (I)

Consult with the dietitian (I)

Communication
  Provide knowledge regarding the causes of hypermagnesium (I)
  Listen to the patient's concerns, fears, and anxieties (I)
  Reduce the patient's anxiety level (I)

Activity
  Encourage alternative rest and moderate activity periods (I)
  Provide diversional activity (I)
  Evaluate any alteration in the patient's thought process (I)

Pain
  Ask the patient what makes him or her comfortable (I)
  Evaluate the type, location, and duration of pain (I)

Bibliography
Krupp, M., Chalton, M., & Werdegar, D. *Current medical diagnoses and treatment.* Los Altos, Calif.: Lange Medical Publications, 1985.

TISSUE PERFUSION, ALTERATION IN
Renal Tissue Perfusion, Decreased

DEFINITION
Decreased renal tissue perfusion implies a reduction in blood flow through the glomerularized peritubular capillaries.

ETIOLOGY
  Renal artery stenosis
  Trauma
  Shock
  Decreased cardiac output
  Hypotension
  Acute tubular necrosis
  Renal failure

DEFINING CHARACTERISTICS

Regulatory Behaviors
  Edema
  Oliguria
  Increased CVP

Increased PAP
Increased PCWP
Dyspnea
Fatigue
Pallor
Tachycardia
Pain

Cognitive Behaviors
Confusion
Anxiety
Irritability
Apprehension

NURSING RESPONSIBILITIES

Assessment

Assess regulatory behaviors indicative of decreased renal tissue perfusion (I)

Assess cognitive behaviors indicative of decreased renal tissue perfusion (I)

Monitor the ECG pattern continuously (I)

Observe the side or therapeutic effects of prescribed medications (I)

Auscultate the femoral artery for bruits (I)

Inspect the jugular veins (I)

Inspect the skin for edema (I)

Inspect the skin for pallor (I)

Auscultate the chest for abnormal breath sounds (I)

Auscultate the chest for adventitious breath sounds (I)

Interventions

Fluid

Administer prescribed medications (D)

Restrict fluid intake, based upon the amount of urinary volume (ID)

Evaluate serum electrolytes, BUN, and creatinine (I)

Measure intake and output (I)

Weigh the patient (I)

Evaluate data from hemodynamic parameters: CVP, PAP, PCWP, SVR, and CO (I)

Measure arterial blood pressure and MAP (I)

Aeration

Provide oxygen via mask, nasal catheter, or nasal prongs at the prescribed percentage and flow rate (D)

Evaluate the patient's breathing pattern for shortness of breath or dyspnea (I)

Evaluate arterial blood gasses (I)

Nutrition

Consult with the dietitian (I)

Provide knowledge regarding dietary restrictions appropriate to the patient's illness (I)

Communication

Instruct the patient about diagnostic procedures (ID)

Evaluate any alteration in the patient's thought process (I)

Listen to the patient's concerns and fears (I)

Provide knowledge regarding the causes of decreased renal tissue perfusion (I)

Support the patient through diagnostic procedures (I)

Activity

Encourage the use of diversional activities (I)

Provide rest periods between interventions (I)

Encourage moderate activity (I)

Pain

Administer prescribed medications for pain (D)

Evaluate for the presence of pain (I)

Bibliography

Carpenito, L. J. *Handbook of nursing diagnosis.* Philadelphia: Lippincott, 1984.

Gettrust, K., Ryan, S. & Engleman, D. *Applied nursing diagnosis.* New York: Wiley, 1985.

Kim, M. J., McFarland, G., & McLane, A. *Nursing diagnosis.* St. Louis: C. V. Mosby, 1984.

URINARY ELIMINATION, ALTERATION IN PATTERNS OF

Urinary Output, Decreased, Oliguria

DEFINITION

Oliguria is defined as urinary volume less than 10 mL/hr (0.2 mL/min).

ETIOLOGY
Dehydration
Shock
Fever
Increased ADH
Acute renal failure
Acute tubular necrosis
Malignant nephrosclerosis
Glomerulonephritis
Malignant hypertension
Pyelonephritis

DEFINING CHARACTERISTICS

Regulatory Behaviors
Change in the pattern of urinary volume
Dark, amber urine
High specific gravity
Edema

Cognitive Behaviors
Irritability
Anxiety
Restlessness
Apprehension

NURSING RESPONSIBILITIES

Assessment
Assess regulatory behaviors associated with oliguria (I)
Assess cognitive behaviors associated with oliguria (I)
Observe the side or therapeutic effects of prescribed medications (I)
Assess the patient's neurological status (I)
Inspect the urine color and for the presence of precipitates (I)
Auscultate the heart for rate, rhythm, and regularity (I)
Inspect for edema (I)
Inspect the neck for vein distension (I)
Auscultate the chest for adventitious breath sounds (I)

Interventions

Fluid

Administer prescribed IV fluids (D)

Measure urinary volume q1h (I)

Measure specific gravity as necessary (I)

Provide Foley care (I)

Measure all fluid intake (I)

Evaluate serum electrolytes, BUN, and creatinine (I)

Aeration

Provide oxygen at the prescribed percentage and flow rate (D)

Reduce meaningless environmental stimuli (I)

Evaluate arterial blood gasses (I)

Nutrition

Encourage the patient to eat the prescribed diet (I)

Limit the patient's daily fluid intake according to renal status and daily output (I)

Communication

Listen to the patient's concerns and fears (I)

Reduce the patient's anxiety level (I)

Inform the physician of any changes in the patient's condition (I)

Provide knowledge regarding the causes of oliguria (I)

Provide knowledge regarding the purposes of diagnostic procedures (I)

Activity

Evaluate any alterations in the patient's thought process (I)

Encourage alternative rest and moderate activity periods (I)

Provide diversional activities (I)

Reduce the demand for cognitive functioning when the patient is ill or fatigued (I)

Pain

Administer prescribed medications (D)

Discuss possible pain-relieving measures (I)

Evaluate the type, location, and duration of pain (I)

Bibliography

Carpenito, L. J. *Handbook of nursing diagnosis.* Philadelphia: Lippincott, 1984.

Gettrust, K., Ryan, S., & Engleman, D. *Applied nursing diagnosis.* New York: Wiley 1985.

Kim, M. J., McFarland, G., & McLane, A. *Nursing diagnosis.* St. Louis: C. V. Mosby, 1984.

Urinary Output, Increased, Polyuria

DEFINITION

Polyuria is defined as urinary volume greater than 1200 mL/hr (20 mL/min).

ETIOLOGY

  Depressed ADH
  Diabetes insipidus
  Neurogenic diabetes insipidus
  Diabetes mellitus
  Diuretics
  Onset of severe hypertension
  Post-obstructive diuresis following relief of obstruction
  Infusion of hypotonic saline

DEFINING CHARACTERISTICS

Regulatory Behaviors

  Increased urinary volume
  Pale urine
  Nocturia
  Low specific gravity
  Thirst
  Dry skin
  Weight loss

Cognitive Behaviors

  Expression of urinary frequency
  Altered sleep pattern
  Irritability

NURSING RESPONSIBILITIES

Assessment

Assess regulatory behaviors associated with polyuria (I)

Assess cognitive behaviors associated with polyuria (I)

Observe the side or therapeutic effects of prescribed medications (I)

Auscultate the chest for adventitious breath sounds (I)

Interventions

Fluid

Administer prescribed medications (D)

Administer prescribed IV fluids (D)

Evaluate the skin for color, temperature, and turgor (I)

Measure intake, urinary volume, and specific gravity (I)

Measure blood pressure and MAP (I)

Evaluate serum electrolytes, BUN, and creatinine levels (I)

Evaluate the color of urinary output (I)

Aeration

Evaluate arterial blood gasses (I)

Reduce unnecessary environmental stimuli (I)

Nutrition

Encourage the patient to eat the prescribed diet (I)

Consult with the dietitian (I)

Communication

Listen to the patient's concerns regarding increased urinary frequency (I)

Reduce the patient's anxiety level (I)

Inform the physician of any changes in the patient's urinary volume (I)

Activity

Encourage alternative rest and moderate activity periods (I)

Evaluate any alteration in the patient's thought process (I)

Provide or encourage diversional activities (I)

Pain

Administer the prescribed analgesics (D)

Evaluate for the presence of pain upon urination (I)

Evaluate for the frequency of pain (I)

Bibliography
Carpenito, L. J. *Handbook of nursing diagnosis.* Philadelphia: Lippin-
cott, 1984.
Gettrust, K., Ryan, S., & Engleman, D. *Applied nursing diagnosis.* New
York: Wiley, 1985.
Kim, M. J., McFarland, G., & McLane, A. *Nursing diagnosis.* St. Louis:
C. V. Mosby, 1984.

URINARY ELIMINATION, ALTERATION IN PATTERN OF
Urinary Incontinence

DEFINITION
Urinary incontinence is a condition characterized by the involuntary escape of urine from the lower urinary tract in a
degree that imposes a social or hygienically unacceptable situation upon the individual (Hald, 1975).

ETIOLOGY
Impairment of the nerve pathway to the bladder
    Autonomic neurogenic bladder
        Damage to lower portion of the spinal cord due to
            Trauma
            Congenital abnormalities
    Reflex neurogenic bladder
        Damage to the spinal cord between the cortical and
            the sacral bladder centers
    Atonic neurogenic bladder
        Damage to the posterior nerve roots, causing retention
            with overflow incontinence
            Diabetic neuropathy
    Uninhibited neurogenic bladder
        Bladder center in the cerebral cortex is damaged
            CVA
            Parkinsonism
Dysfunction of the bladder or urethra
    Acute cystitis
    Urinary tract infection (UTI)
    Carcinoma

Fecal impaction and prostatic enlargement
Alteration in the pelvic diaphragm
    Uterine prolapse
    Cystocele
    Rectocele
Metabolic abnormalities
    Hypokalemia
    Hypercalcemia
    Hyperglycemia
Psychological factors
    Confusion
    Disorientation
    Stress

DEFINING CHARACTERISTICS

Regulatory Behaviors
Incontinence
Constant dribbling
Decreased force of stream
Distended or palpable bladder
Dysuria
Frequency
Nocturia
Anuria
Urgency
Burning
Cloudy urine
Loss of urine in standing position

COGNITIVE BEHAVIORS
Unaware of incontinence
Confusion
Sensation of bladder fullness
Anxiousness

NURSING RESPONSIBILITIES

Assessment
Assess regulatory behaviors indicative of urinary incontinence (I)
Assess cognitive behaviors indicative of urinary incontinence (I)

Assess for degree of urgency, frequency of urination, amount of urination, and amount of incontinence (I)

Assess the bladder's ability to contract by asking the patient to void (I)

Assess the patient's ability to sense the need to void (I)

Monitor the bladder distension and the ability to void (I)

Monitor the signs and symptoms of a UTI (I)

Interventions

Fluid

Administer prescribed medications (D)

Measure intake, output, and specific gravity (I)

Monitor the patency of indwelling catheters (I)

Evaluate the urine for changes in color (I)

Evaluate laboratory data: electrolytes, BUN, and creatinine levels (I)

Encourage fluid intake to avoid bladder infection (I)

Aeration

Reduce meaningless environmental stimuli (I)

Communication

Support the patient's attempt to follow the bladder training program (I)

Encourage the patient to limit fluid prior to bedtime (I)

Reinforce the wellness role, such as maintaining independence (I)

Encourage the patient to verbalize concerns and frustration when incontinence occurs (I)

Keep teaching on a simple level (I)

Activity

Provide sanitary napkins or protective pants during the day (I)

Encourage diversional activity (I)

Pain

Administer prescribed medications (I)

Evaluate the type, location, and duration of pain (I)

Bibliography

De Rosa, S. Urinary incontinence. In Jacobs, M. & Geels, W. (eds.), *Signs and Symptoms in Nursing*. Philadelphia: Lippincott, 1985, pp. 404–420.

Hald, T. Problems of urinary incontinence. In Cadwell, K. (ed.): *Urinary Incontinence*, New York: Grune & Stratton, 1975.

Gettrust, K., Ryan, S., and Engleman, D. *Applied Nursing Diagnosis*. New York: Wiley, 1985.

ACID-BASE IMBALANCE
Acid-Base Imbalance, Metabolic Acidosis

DEFINITION

Metabolic acidosis is defined as an increase in hydrogen-ion concentration and a decrease in pH.

ETIOLOGY

Bicarbonate loss
    Proximal renal tubular acidosis
    Dilutional acidosis
    Carbonic anhydrase inhibitors
    Primary hyperparathyroidism
    Diarrheal states
    Small-bowel drainage
    Ureterosigmoidostomy
Failure of bicarbonate regeneration
    Distal, gradient-limited renal tubular acidosis
    Hyporeninemic hypoaldosteronism
    Diuretics
        Triamterene
        Spironolactone
    Acidifying salts
        Ammonium chloride
        Lysine hydrochloride
        Arginine hydrochloride
        Hyperalimentation
    Reduced excretion of inorganic acids
        Renal failure
Accumulation of organic acids
    Lactic acidosis
    Ketoacidosis
        Alcoholism
        Diabetes
        Starvation

Ingestion
Salicylates
Paraldehyde
Methanol
Ethylene glycol

DEFINING CHARACTERISTICS
Regulatory Behaviors
Hyperpnea
Decrease total CO_2
Increased potassium
Increased pulse
Increased chloride
Cognitive Behaviors
Mental alertness, unless acidosis is severe
Lethargy
Apprehension

NURSING RESPONSIBILITIES
Assessment
Assess regulatory behaviors indicative of metabolic acidosis (I)
Assess cognitive behaviors indicative of metabolic acidosis (I)
Monitor the ECG pattern continuously (I)
Assess the patient's neurological status (I)
Observe the side or therapeutic effects of prescribed medications (I)
Auscultate the heart for abnormal heart sounds (I)
Auscultate the heart for rate, rhythm, and regularity (I)
Inspect the jugular veins (I)
Inspect the skin for edema (I)
Auscultate the chest for adventitious breath sounds (I)
Auscultate the chest for respiratory rate, rhythm, and regularity (I)
Inspect the patient for cyanosis (I)
Palpate the chest for a precordial heave (I)
Percuss the chest for abnormal resonance (I)
Percuss the posterior chest for decreased diaphragmatic descent (I)

Inspect the abdomen for ascites (I)
Inspect the abdomen for distension (I)

Interventions

Fluid

Administer appropriate IV fluids (D)
Administer prescribed medications (D)
Administer $NaHCO_3$ to reverse severe acidosis (D)
Check for the presence/absence of peripheral pulses and for bilateral equality (I)
Measure arterial blood pressure and MAP (I)
Regulate the IV flow rate and check for patency (I)
Evaluate data from hemodynamic parameters: PAP, PCWP, CVP, SVR, and CO (I)
Inform the physician of changes in hemodynamic status (I)
Measure intake and output (I)
Weigh the patient (I)
Evaluate the skin for color, temperature, and diaphoresis (I)
Evaluate laboratory studies (I)

Aeration

Administer humidified oxygen by mask, nasal prongs, or nasal catheter at the prescribed percentage and flow rate (D)
Maintain adequate ventilation through the use of continuous ventilatory support (D)
Evaluate the breathing pattern for dyspnea (I)
Obtain arterial blood gasses from an arterial line (I)
Evaluate arterial blood gasses (I)
Encourage the patient to cough, turn, and deep-breathe (I)
Reduce extraneous environmental stimuli (I)

Nutrition

Encourage the patient to maintain the prescribed diet (I)
Assist the patient with eating (I)
Adjust the patient's diet to his or her needs and lifestyle (I)
Review dietary intake with the patient to determine his or her level of adherence to the prescribed diet (I)

Communication

Listen to the patient's concerns, fears, and anxieties (I)
Reduce the patient's anxiety level (I)

Inform the physician of any changes in the patient's condition (I)

Encourage decision making (I)

Provide knowledge regarding the causes of metabolic acidosis (I)

Activity

Change the patient's position q2h (I)

Encourage alternate rest and moderate activity periods (I)

Reduce the demand for cognitive functioning when the patient is ill or fatigued (I)

Provide diversional activities (I)

Pain

Discuss possible pain-relieving measures (I)

Evaluate the type, location, and duration of pain (I)

Prepare the patient for a painful experience (I)

Bibliography

Wyngaarden, J. & Smith, L. *Cecil textbook of medicine* (17th ed.). Philadelphia: W. B. Saunders, 1985.

Acid Base Imbalance, Metabolic Alkalosis

DEFINITION

Metabolic alkalosis is defined as a decrease in hydrogen-ion concentration and an increase in pH.

ETIOLOGY

Extracellular fluid (ECF) volume contraction

Potassium depletion

Increased distal salt delivery

Mineralocorticoid excess

Liddle's syndrome

Bicarbonate loading

   Posthypercapneic alkalosis

Delayed conversion of administered organic acids

Prolonged nasogastric suction

DEFINING CHARACTERISTICS

Regulatory Behaviors

Hypopnea

Positive Trousseau's sign

Positive Chvostek's sign
Hyperactive deep-tendon reflexes
Muscle spasm
Arrhythmias
Muscle weakness
Increased total CO_2
Decreased potassium
Decreased pulse
Decreased chloride

Cognitive Behaviors
Somnolence
Obtundation
Coma

NURSING RESPONSIBILITIES

Assessment
Assess regulatory behaviors indicative of metabolic alkalosis
(I)
Assess cognitive behaviors indicative of metabolic alkalosis
(I)
Monitor the ECG pattern continuously (I)
Observe the side or therapeutic effects of prescribed medications (I)
Assess the patient's neurological status (I)
Auscultate the heart for abnormal heart sounds (I)
Inspect the skin for cyanosis (I)
Auscultate the chest for abnormal breath sounds (I)

Interventions

Fluid
Provide adequate parenteral intake, including electrolytes
(D)
Administer prescribed medications (D)
Dilute hydrochloric acid
Lysine hydrochloride
Arginine hydrochloride
Potassium chloride
Check for the presence/absence of peripheral pulses and for
bilateral equality (I)

Measure arterial blood pressure and MAP (I)

Evaluate data from hemodynamic parameters: PAP, PCWP, CVP, SVR, and CO (I)

Measure intake and output (I)

Evaluate laboratory studies (I)

Aeration

Provide oxygen at the prescribed percentage and flow rate (D)

Evaluate the patient's breathing pattern for shortness of breath and dyspnea (I)

Evaluate arterial blood gasses (I)

Reduce extraneous environmental stimuli (I)

Nutrition

Restrict the patient's sodium intake to prevent renal potassium wasting (D)

Assist the patient with eating (I)

Encourage the patient to eat the prescribed diet (I)

Communication

Reduce the patient's anxiety level (I)

Encourage self-performance (I)

Keep teaching on a simple-to-complex level, depending upon the patient (I)

Provide knowledge regarding the causes of metabolic alkalosis (I)

Activity

Encourage alternate rest and moderate activity periods (I)

Inspect for muscle spasms and hyperactive reflexes (I)

Supervise the patient's initial ambulation so as to prevent falling due to muscle weakness (I)

Evaluate any alterations in the patient's thought process (I)

Pain

Discuss possible pain-relieving measures (I)

Evaluate the type, location, and duration of pain (I)

Prepare the patient for a painful experience (I)

Bibliography

Krupp, M., Chatton, M., & Werdeger, D. *Current medical diagnosis and treatment.* Los Altos, Calif.: Lange Medical Publications, 1985.

Wyngaarden, J. & Smith, L. *Cecil textbook of medicine* (17th ed.). Philadelphia: W. B. Saunders, 1985.

GASTROINTESTINAL SYSTEM

As with other systems, the critical care nurse applies his or her knowledge of the functions of the gastrointestinal system. The nurse also incorporates data collected from inspection, auscultation, percussion, and palpation into the collaborative nursing diagnosis.

FLUID VOLUME DEFICIT

Actual Fluid Volume and Electrolyte Deficit, Diabetic Shock

DEFINITION
Diabetic shock is characterized by metabolic acidosis and severe dehydration of the vascular, interstitial, and intracellular fluid compartments.

ETIOLOGY
  Diabetes mellitus
  Insulin deficit
  Malnutrition
  Lack of compliance with diet
  Diabetic acidosis

DEFINING CHARACTERISTICS

Regulatory Behaviors
  Emaciation
  Dry skin
  Thirst
  Visual disturbances
  Dizziness
  Weakness
  Kussmaul's respiration
  Polyuria
  Anorexia
  Headache

Abdominal pain
Nausea
Vomiting

Cognitive Behaviors
Drowsiness
Listlessness
Unconsciousness
Excitement
Delirium

NURSING RESPONSIBILITIES

Assessment

Assess regulatory behaviors indicative of diabetic shock (I)
Assess cognitive behaviors indicative of diabetic shock (I)
Monitor the ECG pattern continuously (I)
Observe the side or therapeutic effects of prescribed medications (I)
Auscultate the heart for rate, rhythm, and regularity (I)
Palpate for arterial pulsations and/or peripheral pulses (I)
Inspect the skin for pallor or cyanosis (I)
Inspect for Kussmaul's respiration (I)
Auscultate the chest for abnormal breath sounds (I)

Interventions

Fluid

Administer appropriate IV fluids and electrolytes (D)
Administer prescribed medications (D)
Insulin
Evaluate for dehydration (I)
Evaluate the skin for color, temperature, dryness, and turgor (I)
Measure blood pressure and MAP (I)
Measure intake, output, and specific gravity (I)
Weigh the patient (I)
Evaluate serum electrolytes, BUN, creatinine, and glucose levels (I)

Aeration

Provide oxygen at the prescribed percentage and flow rate (D)

Evaluate the breathing pattern for shortness of breath or dyspnea (I)

Evaluate for airway obstruction (I)

Establish and maintain a patent airway (I)

Nutrition

Adjust the diabetic diet to the patient's lifestyle (ID)

Encourage the patient to maintain the prescribed diabetic diet (I)

Consult with the dietitian (I)

Review the dietary intake with the patient to determine his or her level of adherence to the prescribed diet (I)

Communication

Provide knowledge regarding the causes of diabetic shock (I)

Encourage patient self-performance (I)

Encourage the acceptance of self-limitations (I)

Encourage decision making (I)

Listen to the patient's concerns and fears (I)

Inform the physician of any changes in the patient's condition (I)

Arrange situations that encourage the patient's autonomy (I)

Inform the patient as to what is expected of him or her in critical care (I)

Activity

Evaluate the patient's ability to ambulate without supervision (I)

Evaluate the patient's activity tolerance (I)

Provide rest periods between nursing interventions (I)

Evaluate any alterations in the patient's thought process (I)

Evaluate any alterations in consciousness (I)

Inspect the eyes for pupil size, equality, and response to light (I)

Pain

Administer prescribed medications (D)

Ask the patient what makes him or her comfortable (I)

Reduce physical discomfort that could interfere with cognitive structure (I)

Evaluate the type and location of pain (I)

Bibliography

Bordicks, K. *Patterns of shock implications for nursing care* (2nd ed.). New York: Macmillan, 1980.

Borg, N., Nikas, D., Stark, J., & Williams, S. *Core curriculum for critical care nursing.* Philadelphia: W. B. Saunders, 1981.

BOWEL ELIMINATION, ALTERATION IN
Bowel Elimination, Decreased, Constipation

DEFINITION
Constipation is defined as a decreased frequency of bowel movements in relation to normal elimination patterns.

ETIOLOGY
    Fear of painful defecation
    Prolonged bed rest
    Spasm of the anus due to inflamed hemorrhoids
    Ulcerated fissure
    Chronic use of enemas
    Diet low in roughage
    Medication
    Neuromuscular impairment
    Musculoskeletal impairment
    Diagnostic procedures
    Pregnancy
    Inactivity
    Weak abdominal musculature
    Inadequate fluid intake
    Pain during defecation

DEFINING CHARACTERISTICS

Regulatory Behaviors
    Hard-formed stool
    Palpable mass
    Straining at stool
    Decreased bowel sounds
    Less than the usual amount of stool
    Nausea
    Abdominal pain

    Back pain
    Headache
    Use of laxatives
    Reported feeling of pressure in rectum

Cognitive Behaviors
    Sensation of abdominal fullness
    Desire to defecate
    Listlessness

NURSING RESPONSIBILITIES

Assessment

    Assess regulatory behaviors indicative of constipation (I)
    Assess cognitive behaviors indicative of constipation (I)
    Observe the side or therapeutic effects of prescribed medications (I)
    Assess the patient's prehospital diet and bowel habits (I)
    Inspect the stool for color, consistency, and amount (I)
    Auscultate the chest for respiratory rate, rhythm, and regularity (I)
    Inspect the abdomen for distension (I)
    Palpate the abdomen for tenderness, rigidity, and masses (I)

Interventions

Fluid

    Administer prescribed stool softener (D)
    Administer prescribed enema(s) (ID)
    Provide adequate fluids in the diet (I)
    Provide juices that might stimulate bowel elimination (I)
    Measure urinary volume and specific gravity (I)
    Regulate the IV fluid and check for patency (I)
    Evaluate laboratory studies: serum electrolytes, BUN, creatinine, and urinalysis (I)
    Evaluate the skin for dryness and turgor (I)
    Provide a bedside commode, not a bedpan, as tolerated (I)
    Record the color, consistency, amount, and odor of all stool (I)
    Evaluate the patient's fluid balance to determine whether or not fluid restriction is too severe (I)
    Review with the pharmacist drugs that may cause constipation (I)

Aeration

Administer humidified oxygen by mask, nasal cannula, or nasal prongs at the prescribed percentage and flow rate (D)

Reduce excessive and/or meaningless environmental stimuli (I)

Nutrition

Consult with both dietitian and physician regarding the patient's diet (I)

Encourage the inclusion of roughage foods in the diet (I)

Instruct the patient regarding foods high in bulk and residue (I)

Long-fibered vegetables
Celery
Cabbage
Greens
Raw fruits with skins
Raw or cooked fruits
Prunes
Apricots
Figs
Dates

Adjust the diet to the patient's lifestyle (I)

Communication

Reduce the patient's anxiety level (I)

Listen to the patient's concerns regarding his or her bowel problem and possible causes (I)

Encourage patient self-performance

Instruct the patient regarding the causes of constipation, such as diet, medications, or inactivity (I)

Instruct the patient to respond to the elimination urge (I)

Activity

Encourage moderate physical activity (I)

Assist the patient in establishing a pattern of elimination (I)

Allow adequate time to use the bathroom or commode (I)

Provide the patient with privacy (I)

Inspect for abnormal body movement (I)

Measure abdominal girth and fluid wave (I)

Pain
   Administer analgesics as prescribed (D)
   Discuss possible pain-relieving measures (I)
   Reassure the patient that pain will subside or be relieved (I)
   Evaluate the type, location, and degree of pain (I)

Bibliography

Carpenito, L. J. *Handbook of nursing diagnosis.* Philadelphia: Lippincott, 1984.
Gettrust, K., Ryan, S., & Engleman, D. *Applied nursing diagnosis.* New York: Wiley, 1985.
Kim, M. J., McFarland, G., & McLane, A. *Nursing diagnosis.* St. Louis: C. V. Mosley, 1984.

Bowel Elimination, Increased, Diarrhea

DEFINITION
Diarrhea is defined as an increase in frequency, fluidity, and/or volume of stool in relation to the patient's normal elimination patterns.

ETIOLOGY
   Anxiety
   Viral infections
      Enterovirus
      Rotavirus
   Bacterial infections
      Campylobacter jejuni
      Shigella
      Salmonella
      Yersinia enterocolitica
   Bacterial toxins
      Clostridium difficile
      Escherichia coli
      Staphylococcus
      Vibrio parahaemolutieus
      Vibrio cholerae
   Parasitic infections
      Giardia lamblia
      Entamoeba hystytica

    Cryptosporidium
    Isospora
Fecal impaction
Antibiotic therapy
Inflammatory bowel disease
Catharsis habituation
Vagotomy
Carcinoma
Gastrocolic fistula
Hepatitis
Bile duct obstruction
Primary small-bowel mucosal diseases
Intestinal blind loop syndrome
Pancreatic endocrine tumors
Pelvic disease
Tabes dorsalis
Diabetic neuropathy
Hyperthyroidism
IgA deficiency
Marasmus
Kwashiorkor
Excessive intake of fresh fruit

DEFINING CHARACTERISTICS

Regulatory Behaviors
Abdominal pain
Cramping
Change in the color of stools
Increased fluidity of stool
Increased volume of stool
Weight loss
Foul-smelling stool
Urgency
Fever
Fatigue
Anorexia

Cognitive Behaviors
Irritability
Apprehension

Tiredness
Lassitude
Confusion

NURSING RESPONSIBILITIES

Assessment

Assess regulatory behaviors indicative of diarrhea (I)
Assess cognitive behaviors indicative of diarrhea (I)
Observe the side or therapeutic effects of prescribed medications (I)
Assess the patient's prehospital experiences with diarrhea (I)
Auscultate the chest for respiratory rate, rhythm, and regularity (I)
Auscultate the abdomen for abnormal bowel sounds (I)
Palpate the abdomen for tenderness, rigidity, and masses (I)

Interventions

Fluid

Obtain a stool specimen for ovium and parasite testing (D)
Administer prescribed medications (D)
    Pepto-Bismol
    Narcotic analogs
    Lomotil
    Loperamide (Imodium)
    Paregoric
    Codeine phosphate
Administer prescribed parenteral fluids (D)
Measure the amount of diarrheal output (I)
Record the odor, color, and frequency of stool (I)
Measure urinary output and specific gravity (I)
Evaluate serum electrolyte studies (I)
Weigh the patient daily (I)
Test the patient's stool for occult blood (I)
Regulate the IV flow rate and check for patency (I)

Aeration

Administer humidified oxygen by mask, nasal prongs, or nasal catheter at the prescribed percentage and flow rate (D)
Evaluate the skin for color changes (I)

Nutrition

Provide small, soft feedings (D)

Administer total parenteral nutrition (D)

Consult with both dietitian and physician regarding the patient's diet (I)

Provide knowledge regarding the patient's diet (I)

Instruct the patient to eliminate foods that contribute to his or her diarrhea (I)

Communication

Reduce the patient's anxiety level (I)

Listen to the patient's concerns, fears, or anxieties (I)

Encourage patient to participation in self-care (I)

Activity

Reduce the demand for cognitive functioning when the patient is ill or fatigued (I)

Encourage alternate rest and activity periods (I)

Provide diversional activities (I)

Pain

Administer analgesics as prescribed (D)

Evaluate the type, location, and duration of pain (I)

Ask the patient what makes him or her comfortable (I)

Bibliography

Carpenito, L. J. *Handbook of nursing diagnosis.* Philadelphia: Lippincott, 1984.

Gettrust, K., Ryan, S., & Engleman, D. *Applied nursing diagnosis.* New York: Wiley, 1985.

Kim, M. J., McFarland, G., & McLane, A. *Nursing diagnosis.* St. Louis: C. V. Mosby, 1984.

Bowel Elimination, Uncontrolled, Incontinence

DEFINITION

Anal incontinence is the involuntary loss of rectal contents.

ETIOLOGY

Obstetric tears

Anorectal operations

Fistulotomy

Sphincterotomy
Hemorrhoidectomy
Rectal prolapse repair
Postvagotomy
Ileorectal anastamosis
Neurological disturbances
Tabes dorsalis
Multiple sclerosis
Organic brain syndrome (Alzheimer's disease)
Neurogenic bowel

DEFINING CHARACTERISTICS

Regulatory Behaviors
Involuntary passage of stool
Discomfort
Abdominal cramps
Fatigue

Cognitive Behaviors
Feeling of urgency
Apprehension
Uneasiness
Restlessness

NURSING RESPONSIBILITIES

Assessment
Assess regulatory behaviors indicative of anal incontinence (I)
Assess cognitive behaviors indicative of anal incontinence (I)

Interventions

Fluid
Administer prescribed medications (D)
Administer prescribed IV fluids (D)
Provide a commode 30 min after eating (I)
Measure or estimate the amount of stool incontinence (I)
Measure urinary output and specific gravity (I)
Evaluate serum electrolyte studies (I)
Record the odor, color, and frequency of stool (I)
Evaluate the skin for color, temperature, and turgor (I)

Aeration

Administer humidified oxygen via nasal catheter, mask, or nasal prongs at the prescribed percentage and flow rate (D)

Evaluate the skin for pallor or cyanosis (I)

Eliminate extraneous environmental stimuli (I)

Nutrition

Provide knowledge regarding the patient's diet (I)

Consult with both dietitian and physician regarding the patient's diet (I)

Review dietary intake with the patient to determine his or her level of adherence to the prescribed diet (I)

Communication

Provide knowledge regarding the causes of incontinence (I)

Reduce the patient's anxiety level (I)

Listen to the patient's concerns, fears, or anxieties regarding incontinence (I)

Activity

Palplate the abdomen for tenderness, rigidity, and masses (I)

Reduce the demand for cognitive functioning when the patient is ill or fatigued (I)

Encourage alternate rest and moderate activity periods (I)

Provide diversional activity (I)

Evaluate any alteration in the patient's thought process (I)

Encourage the use of a toilet, commode, or bedpan before physical activity (I)

Pain

Administer analgesics as prescribed (D)

Ask the patient what makes him or her comfortable (I)

Bibliography

Carpenito, L. J. *Handbook of nursing diagnosis.* Philadelphia: Lippincott, 1984.

Gettrust, K., Ryan, S., & Engleman, D. *Applied nursing diagnosis.* New York: Wiley, 1985.

Kim, M. J., McFarland, G., & McLane, A. *Nursing diagnosis.* St. Louis: C. V. Mosby, 1984.

FLUID VOLUME EXCESS

Extracellular Fluid Volume Excess, Intraperitoneal Edema or Ascites

DEFINITION
Ascites is the accumulation of serous fluid in the abdominal cavity.

ETIOLOGY
Hepatic cirrhosis
Pancreatitis
Malignancy
Hypoproteinemia
Portal hypertension
Chronic heart failure
Constrictive pericarditis
Myxedema

DEFINING CHARACTERISTICS
Regulatory Behaviors
Increased abdominal girth
Weight gain
Pleural effusion
Edema
    Peripheral
    Ankle
    Presacral
Presence of fluid wave
Percussion dullness of the flanks in the supine position

Cognitive Behaviors
Irritability
Anxiety
Apprehension
Confusion
Lethargy

NURSING RESPONSIBILITIES
Assessment
Assess regulatory behaviors indicative of ascites (I)
Assess cognitive behaviors indicative of ascites (I)

Monitor the ECG pattern continuously (I)

Observe the side or therapeutic effects of prescribed medications (I)

Auscultate the heart for abnormal heart sounds (I)

Auscultate the heart for rate, rhythm, and regularity (I)

Inspect the jugular veins for distension (I)

Palpate the chest for thrill (I)

Palpate the chest for an abnormal precordial thrust (I)

Percuss the chest for abnormal resonance (I)

Inspect the abdomen for intraperitoneal edema or ascites (I)

Inspect the abdomen for vein engorgement (I)

Palpate the abdomen for tenderness or masses (I)

Interventions

Fluid

Administer the prescribed medications (D)
  Aldactone
  Dyrenium
  Zaroxolyn
  Lasix

Assist the physician with paracentesis (D)

Evaluate laboratory studies: liver panel, electrolytes, BUN, creatinine, and CBC (I)

Evaluate data from hemodynamic parameters: PAP, PCWP, CVP, SVR, and CO (I)

Evaluate peripheral pulses and check for equality (I)

Evaluate the skin for color, temperature, and diaphoresis (I)

Measure urinary volume and specific gravity (I)

Measure oral and parenteral fluid intake (I)

Restrict fluid intake (I)

Measure arterial blood pressure and MAP (I)

Measure the amount of nasogastric drainage (I)

Aeration

Administer mechanical ventilation (D)

Administer humidified oxygen by mask, nasal cannula, or nasal prongs at the prescribed percentage and flow rate (D)

Evaluate arterial blood gasses (I)

Evaluate the patient's breathing pattern for dyspnea or shortness of breath (I)

Reduce meaningless environmental stimuli (I)

Suction the patient as necessary (I)

Nutrition

> Provide the patient with the prescribed diet (D)
>
> Restrict the patient's sodium intake (D)
>
> Consult with both physician and dietitian regarding the patient's diet (I)

Communication

> Reduce the patient's anxiety level (I)
>
> Ask questions that encourage answers reflecting reality perception (I)
>
> Keep teaching on a simple level (I)
>
> Inform the patient regarding what is expected of him or her in critical care (I)
>
> Inform the physician of changes in the patient's condition (I)
>
> Listen to the patient's concerns (I)

Activity

> Change the patient's position q2h (I)
>
> Reduce the demand for cognitive functioning when the patient is ill or fatigued (I)
>
> Encourage the patient to rest (I)
>
> Elevate edematous extremities (I)
>
> Measure the patient's abdominal girth (I)

Pain

> Evaluate the type, location, and duration of pain (I)

Bibliography

Given, B. & Simmons, S. *Gastroenterology in clinical nursing.* St. Louis: C. V. Mosby, 1979.

Roberts, S. *Physiological concepts and the critically ill patient.* Englewood Cliffs, N.J.: Prentice-Hall, 1985, pp. 245–281.

TISSUE PERFUSION, ALTERATION IN

Intra-abdominal Perfusion, Decreased

DEFINITION

Decreased intra-abdominal perfusion implies reduced blood flow through the celiac axis, superior mesenteric artery, or inferior mesenteric artery.

ETIOLOGY
Acute bowel infarction
Mesenteric artery embolism
Nonocclusive intestinal infarction
Ischemic colitis
Mesenteric venous thrombosis
Intramural intestinal hemorrhage
Superior mesenteric artery syndrome
Abdominal angina
Decreased cardiac output
Atrial fibrillation
Trauma

DEFINING CHARACTERISTICS

Regulatory behaviors
Cramping pain
Severe abdominal pain
Hyperactive bowel sounds
Tachycardia
Leukocytosis
Acidosis
Hypotension
Fever
Blood in nasogastric aspirate, vomitus, or stool
Vomiting
Diarrhea

Cognitive Behaviors
Apprehension
Irritability
Fear
Anxiety
Restlessness

NURSING RESPONSIBILITIES

Assessment
Assess regulatory behaviors indicative of decreased intra-
abdominal perfusion (I)
Assess cognitive behaviors indicative of decreased intra-
abdominal perfusion (I)

Monitor the ECG pattern continuously (I)
Observe the side or therapeutic effects of prescribed medications (I)
Inspect the jugular veins for distension (I)
Auscultate the heart for abnormal heart sounds (I)
Auscultate the heart for rate, rhythm, and regularity (I)
Inspect the abdomen for vein engorgement (I)
Palpate the abdomen for tenderness or masses (I)
Palpate the abdominal aorta for increased pulsation (I)
Auscultate the abdomen for abnormal bowel sounds (I)

Interventions

Fluid

Administer prescribed medications (D)
Administer prescribed IV fluids (D)
Evaluate the skin for color, temperature, and diaphoresis (I)
Evaluate data from hemodynamic parameters: PAP, PCWP, CVP, SVR, and CO (I)
Measure urinary volume and specific gravity (I)
Measure arterial blood pressure and MAP (I)

Aeration

Evaluate the breathing pattern for shortness of breath and dyspnea (I)
Evaluate the skin for pallor or cyanosis (I)
Reduce meaningless environmental stimuli (I)

Nutrition

NPO until an abdominal evaluation can be made (D)
Insert nasogastric tube if necessary (ID)
Provide knowledge regarding the purpose of nasogastric tube and food restriction (I)

Communication

Reduce the patient's anxiety level (I)
Inform the physician of any changes in the patient's condition (I)
Listen to the patient's concerns (I)

Activity

Encourage the patient to rest (I)
Change the patient's position q2h (I)

Evaluate any alterations in the patient's thought process (I)
Evaluate the abdomen for distension (I)

Pain

Evaluate for the presence of abdominal pain (I)
Evaluate the location and duration of pain (I)
Reduce the physical discomforts that could interfere with cognitive function (I)
Inform the physician of any sudden expression of abdominal pain (I)

Bibliography

Given, B. & Simmons, S. *Gastroenterology in clinical nursing.* St. Louis: C. V. Mosby, 1979.
Roberts, S. *Physiological concepts and the critically ill patient.* Englewood Cliffs, N.J.: Prentice-Hall, 1985; pp. 245–281.

NUTRITION, ALTERATION IN
Nutritional Alteration, Less Than Body Requirements

DEFINITION

Nutritional intake less than that which meets body requirements implies that an individual loses weight and that the loss is attributed to an inadequate intake of nutrients (rather than a lack of ingestion or absorption of nutrients).

ETIOLOGY

Burns
Infections
Cancer
Trauma
Dysphagia
Crohn's disease
Ileus
Altered sense of taste and/or smell
Anorexia
Nausea
Vomiting
Dyspnea
Fatigue

Depression
Stress
Pain
Increased metabolic rate
Stomatitis
Radiation therapy

DEFINING CHARACTERISTICS

Regulatory behaviors
Weight loss
10 to 20% under ideal weight
Aversion to eating
Thin physique
Reported inadequate food intake
Tachycardia
Activity intolerance
Muscle weakness
Abdominal pain

Cognitive Behaviors
Anxiety
Irritability
Confusion
Apprehension

NURSING RESPONSIBILITIES

Assessment
Assess regulatory behaviors indicative of a nutritional intake providing less than body requirements (I)
Assess cognitive behaviors indicative of nutritional intake providing less than body requirements (I)
Monitor the ECG pattern continuously (I)
Assess the patient's prehospital dietary intake (I)
Inspect skin turgor, mucous membranes, and electrolytes (I)
Auscultate the chest for respiratory rate, rhythm, and regularity (I)

INTERVENTIONS

Fluids
Measure oral, nasogastric, and/or parenteral fluid intake (I)

Measure urinary volume, nasogastric aspirate, vomitus, loose stool, and specific gravity (I)

Evaluate laboratory studies (I)

Serum albumin

Total protein

Serum transferin

Urinary protein

BUN

Creatinine

Provide frequent oral hygiene (I)

Measure blood pressure and MAP (I)

Aeration

Evaluate the breathing pattern for shortness of breath and dyspnea (I)

Reduce meaningless environmental stimuli (I)

Nutrition

Evaluate the amount of dietary intake (I)

Instruct the patient as to what foods are to be eliminated (I)

Provide sufficient fluids with meals (I)

Provide small, frequent feedings (I)

Encourage high-calorie, low-volume supplements between meals (I)

Provide a relaxed atmosphere for eating (I)

Consult with both physician and dietitian (I)

Communication

Inform the physician of any changes in the patient's condition (I)

Provide knowledge regarding the causes of nutritional alteration (I)

Listen to the patient's concerns regarding failure to maintain body weight (I)

Activity

Encourage the patient to use relaxation exercises (I)

Encourage moderate activity when the patient is less fatigued and less weak (I)

Provide periods of rest between nursing interventions (I)

Evaluate any alterations in the patient's thought process (I)

Pain
>   Evaluate for the presence of pain (I)
>   Evaluate the degree of pain experienced (I)
>   Administer analgesics as prescribed (D)

Bibliography

Carpenito, L. J. *Handbook of nursing diagnosis.* Philadelphia: Lippincott, 1984.

Gettrust, K., Ryan, S., & Engleman, D., *Applied nursing diagnosis.* New York: Wiley, 1985.

Kelly, M. *Nursing diagnosis source book: Guidelines for clinical application.* Norwalk, Conn.: Appleton-Century-Crofts, 1985.

Kim, M.J., McFarland, G., & McLane, A. *Nursing diagnosis.* St. Louis: C.V. Mosby, 1984.

Nutritional Alteration, More Than Body Requirements

DEFINITION
Nutritional intake greater than is necessary to meet body requirements or metabolic needs.

ETIOLOGY
>   Appetite-stimulating drugs
>   Inactivity
>   Anxiety
>   Depression
>   Loneliness
>   Boredom
>   Pregnancy
>   Lack of nutritional knowledge
>   Low self-esteem
>   Cultural influences
>   Altered satiety patterns

DEFINING CHARACTERISTICS

Regulatory Behaviors
>   Weight 10–20% over ideal weight
>   Intake in excess of metabolic requirements
>   Triceps skin fold
>   >15 mm in men
>   >25 mm in women

Cognitive Behaviors
Reported undesirable eating patterns
Anxiety
Eating in response to external cues

NURSING RESPONSIBILITIES

Assessment
Assess regulatory behaviors indicative of nutritional intake that is greater than body requirements (I)
Assess cognitive behaviors indicative of nutritional intake that is greater than body requirements (I)
Observe the side or therapeutic effects of prescribed medications (I)
Assess the patient's prehospital eating patterns (I)
Auscultate the heart for rate, rhythm, and regularity (I)

Interventions

Fluid
Administer prescribed medications (D)
Evaluate laboratory studies (I)
Measure intake, urinary volume, and specific gravity (I)
Evaluate the skin for color, temperature, and diaphoresis (I)
Weigh the patient daily (I)

Aeration
Evaluate for dyspnea or shortness of breath upon moderate exertion (I)
Reduce meaningless environmental stimuli (I)

Nutrition
Supplement the patient's diet with vitamins and minerals (D)
Identify with the patient reinforcers for maintaining reduced weight (I)
Facilitate the posthospital development of the patient's individualized plan for weight loss (I)
Provide information regarding the nutritional plan for both patient and family (I)
Encourage the patient to maintain the prescribed diet (I)

Communication
Refer the patient to counseling (D)
Refer the patient to a support group (D)

Inform the patient of the risks of obesity (ID)
Inform the patient of available community resources (I)
Encourage decision making (I)
Encourage the patient to strive toward realistic goals (I)
Explore with the patient previous achievements or successes (I)
Encourage patient acceptance of self-limitations (I)

Activity
Provide alternate rest and moderate activity periods (I)
Change the dependent patient's position q2h (I)
Provide diversional activities (I)
Encourage family members to support the patient in remaining on his or her diet (I)

Pain
Evaluate for the presence of pain (I)
Evaluate the type, location, and duration of pain (I)
Discuss possible pain-relieving measures (I)

Bibliography

Carpenito, L. J. *Handbook of nursing diagnosis.* Philadelphia: Lippincott, 1984.
Gettrust, K., Ryan, S., & Engleman, D. *Applied nursing diagnosis.* New York: Wiley, 1985.
Kelly, M. *Nursing diagnosis source book: Guidelines for clinical application.* Norwalk, Conn.: Appleton-Century-Crofts, 1985.
Kim, M. J., McFarland, G. & McLane, A. *Nursing diagnosis.* St. Louis: C. V. Mosby, 1984.

Swallowing Pattern, Altered, Dysphagia

DEFINITION
Dysphagia is the impaired ability to pass fluids and/or solids through the esophagus.

ETIOLOGY
Benign or malignant esophageal strictures
Hiatal hernia
Trauma
Cricopharyngeal achalasia
Hypertensive cricopharyngeal sphincter

Oropharyngeal dysfunction
Esophageal spasm
Reflux esophagitis
Neuromuscular disease
Edema of the oropharyngeal cavity

DEFINING CHARACTERISTICS

Regulatory Behaviors
Chest pain
Painful swallowing
Weight loss
Malnutrition
Regurgitation of fluids or solids
Decreased gag reflex
Fatigue

Cognitive Behaviors
Apprehension
Fear
Anxiety
Tiredness

NURSING RESPONSIBILITIES

Assessment
Assess regulatory behaviors indicative of dysphagia (I)
Assess cognitive behaviors indicative of dysphagia (I)
Observe the side or therapeutic effects of prescribed medications (I)
Assess the patient's prehospital alteration in swallowing pattern (I)
Inspect the skin for pallor or cyanosis (I)

Interventions

Fluids
Administer prescribed IV fluids (D)
Provide a nasogastric tube for the patient with frequent vomiting (ID)
Measure intake and output (I)
Evaluate for the presence of a gag reflex (I)
Evaluate for regurgitation of foods (I)

Measure vital signs (I)
Evaluate the skin for color, temperature, and the presence of diaphoresis (I)

Aeration
Reduce environmental stimuli (I)
Evaluate the patient's breathing pattern for shortness of breath or dyspnea (I)

Nutrition
Advance the patient's diet as tolerated (ID)
Provide thick or semi-solid fluids (I)
Place food in the back of the mouth on the unaffected side (I)
Administer fluid into the back of the mouth via a large syringe (I)
Reinforce the swallowing sequence (I)
Evaluate for the presence of a gas reflex (I)
Massage the unaffected side of the throat (I)

Communication
Listen to the patient's concerns and fears (I)
Provide knowledge regarding the cause of dysphagia (I)
Instruct the family in ways to support the patient while eating (I)
Reduce the patient's anxiety level (I)

Activity
Provide diversional activities (I)
Encourage and support ambulation (I)

Pain
Provide prescribed analgesics before feeding (D)
Evaluate for the presence of chest pain or pain during swallowing (I)

Bibliography
Gettrust, K., Ryan, S., & Engleman, D. *Applied nursing diagnosis.* New York: Wiley, 1985.
Wyngaarden, J. & Smith, L. *Cecil textbook of medicine* (17th ed.). Philadelphia: W. B. Saunders, 1985.

Oral Mucous Membrane, Alteration In

DEFINITION
An alteration in the oral mucous membrane is defined as a clinical situation in which the patient experiences, or is at risk of developing, disruptions in the oral cavity.

ETIOLOGY
Radiation
Dehydration
Diabetes mellitus
Oral cancer
Infection
Trauma
    Chemical
        Acidic foods
        Drugs
        Alcohol
        Noxious agents
    Mechanical
        Dentures
        Chipped tooth/teeth
        Endotracheal tube
        Surgery
        Nasogastric tube
    Ineffective oral hygiene
    Mouth breathing
    Malnutrition
    Lack of knowledge
    Facial fractures

DEFINING CHARACTERISTICS

Regulatory Behaviors
Coated tongue
Stomatitis
Xerostomia
Oral lesions, tumors, or ulcers
Leukoplakia
Oral pain

Cavities
Halitosis
Hemorrhagic gingivitis

Cognitive Behaviors
Pain
Anxiety
Restlessness

NURSING RESPONSIBILITIES

Assessment

Assess regulatory behaviors indicative of an alteration in the oral mucous membrane (I)
Assess cognitive behaviors indicative of an alteration in the oral mucous membrane (I)
Assess situations contributing to an alteration in the oral mucous membrane (I)

Interventions

Fluid

Measure oral and parenteral intake (I)
Measure output and specific gravity (I)
Encourage oral hygiene (I)
Assist the patient in brushing his or her teeth or dentures (I)

Aeration

Administer oxygen at the prescribed flow rate (D)
Encourage the patient to keep his or her mouth moist while receiving nasal oxygen (I)
Reduce meaningless environmental stimuli (I)

Nutrition

Provide the prescribed diet (ID)
Assist the patient with eating (I)
Provide knowledge regarding toxic or irritating foods (I)

Communication

Instruct the patient regarding the need to avoid smoking and/or alcoholic beverages (I)
Provide knowledge regarding the causes of alteration in the oral mucous membranes (I)

Activity
> Inspect the mouth each day for lesions, ulcers, and/or bleeding (I)
> Encourage the use of diversional activities (I)

Pain
> Administer prescribed analgesics (D)
> Evaluate the type, location, and duration of pain (I)

Bibliography

Carpenito, L. J. *Handbook of nursing diagnosis*. Philadelphia: Lippincott, 1984.

Gettrust, K., Ryan, S., & Engleman, D. *Applied nursing diagnosis*. New York: Wiley, 1985.

Kim, M. J., McFarland, G., & McLane, A. *Nursing diagnosis*. St. Louis: C. V. Mosby, 1984.

INJURY, POTENTIAL FOR
Injury, Blunt Abdominal Trauma

DEFINITION
Blunt abdominal trauma occurs when a force to the abdominal wall causes a diffusion of energy through the abdomen and its contents.

ETIOLOGY
> Automobile accidents
> Industrial accidents
> Home accidents
> Contact sports accidents
> Falls

DEFINING CHARACTERISTICS

Regulatory Behaviors
> Shock
> Change in bowel sounds
> Guaiac-positive specimens for the rectum, bladder, or stomach
> Free air under the diaphragm on kidney, ureter, and bladder (KUB) film

Bruises of the abdominal wall
Crepitus
Tenderness of the abdomen on palpation

Cognitive Behaviors
Restlessness
Agitation
Confusion

NURSING RESPONSIBILITIES

Assessment
Assess regulatory behaviors indicative of blunt abdominal
    trauma (I)
Monitor the ECG pattern continuously (I)
Assess the exact cause of the injury (I)
Auscultate the heart for abnormal heart sounds (I)
Palpate for arterial pulsations/peripheral pulses (I)
Auscultate the heart for rate, rhythm, and regularity (I)
Inspect for cyanosis (I)
Auscultate the abdomen for abnormal bowel sounds (I)
Inspect the abdomen for distension (I)
Palpate the abdomen for tenderness, rigidity, and masses (I)

Interventions

Fluid
Administer prescribed IV fluids (D)
    Ringer's lactate
    Normal saline
Administer prescribed medications (D)
Insert a Foley catheter (ID)
Evaluate urine for abnormal color, content, and odor (I)
Measure intake, urinary volume, and specific gravity (I)
Measure output from the nasogastric tube (I)
Evaluate laboratory studies (I)

Aeration
Administer humidified oxygen (D)
Evaluate the breathing pattern for shortness of breath or
    dyspnea (I)
Evaluate arterial blood gasses (I)
Reduce meaningless environmental stimuli (I)
Maintain an adequate airway (I)

Nutrition
Insert a nasogastric tube (ID)
Provide oral hygiene (I)

Communication
Reduce the patient's anxiety level (I)
Inform the physician of any changes in vital signs or laboratory data (I)
Provide the patient with knowledge regarding treatment procedures and outcomes (I)

Activity
Provide stabilization of the cervical, thoracic, and lumbar spine (D)
Assist the physician with diagnostic tests, such as peritoneal lavage (ID)
Reduce any demand for cognitive functioning when the patient is ill or fatigued (I)

Pain
Administer prescribed medications (D)
Prepare the patient for possible surgery (ID)
Evaluate the type, location, and duration of pain (I)

Bibliography

Budassi, S. & Barber, J. *Mosby's manual of emergency care practices and procedures* (2nd. ed.). St. Louis: C. V. Mosby, 1984.
Sheehy, S. & Barber, J. *Emergency nursing principles and practice* (2nd. ed.). St. Louis: C. V. Mosby, 1985.

Injury, Penetrating Abdominal Trauma

DEFINITION
A penetrating abdominal trauma is the result of a missile or fragment that pierces the abdominal wall and enters the abdominal cavity.

ETIOLOGY
Gunshot wound
Stab wound
Industrial accident

DEFINING CHARACTERISTICS

Regulatory Behaviors
Shock
Hypotension
Tachycardia
Rapid, shallow respiration
Cold, pale, clammy skin

Cognitive Behaviors
Agitation
Restlessness
Confusion
Loss of consciousness

NURSING RESPONSIBILITIES

Assessment
Assess regulatory behaviors indicative of penetrating abdominal trauma (I)
Monitor the ECG pattern continuously (I)
Observe the side or therapeutic effects of prescribed medications (I)
Auscultate the heart for rate, rhythm, and regularity (I)
Auscultate the chest for abnormal breath sounds (I)
Auscultate the chest for respiratory rate, rhythm, and regularity (I)
Inspect the skin for pallor and cyanosis (I)
Inspect the abdomen for the extent of abdominal injuries (I)
Auscultate the abdomen for abnormal bowel sounds (I)
Palpate the area around the wound for tenderness (I)

Interventions

Fluid
Administer prescribed IV fluids (D)
  Ringer's lactate
  Normal saline
Administer prescribed medications (D)
Apply military antishock trousers (MAST) if systolic blood pressure is below 80 mmHg (D)
Apply a wet-to-dry sterile dressing for evisceration (ID)

Insert a Foley catheter (ID)

Insert a nasogastric tube (ID)

Regulate the IV flow rate and check for patency (I)

Measure the patient's blood pressure (I)

Measure intake and output (I)

Evaluate the amount of blood loss through the penetrating wound(s) (I)

Evaluate hemoglobin and hematocrit levels (I)

Aeration

Provide oxygen via mask, nasal catheter, or nasal prongs at the prescribed percentage and flow rate (D)

Evaluate the breathing pattern for dyspnea, tachypnea, or shortness of breath (I)

Evaluate for airway obstruction (I)

Evaluate arterial blood gasses (I)

Nutrition

Connect nasogastric tube to continuous or intermittent suction as prescribed (I)

Provide oral hygiene (I)

Communication

Inform the physician of any changes in the patient's vital signs and laboratory data (I)

Prepare the patient for impending surgery (I)

Prepare the family for the patient's impending surgery (I)

Activity

Utilize a back board and a cervical collar until neck injury is ruled out (D)

Immobilize the patient until the extent of the abdominal injury can be determined (I)

Pain

Administer prescribed analgesics (D)

Evaluate the location of pain (I)

Bibliography

Budassi, S. & Barber, J. *Mosby's manual of emergency care practices and procedures* (2nd ed.). St. Louis: C. V. Mosby, 1984.

Sheehy, S. & Barber, J. *Emergency nursing principles and practice* (2nd ed.). St. Louis: C. V. Mosby, 1985.

INTEGUMENTARY SYSTEM

The appearance of the skin can be a reflection of internal problems. Furthermore, the integumentary system serves as a protective barrier against possible infection. Therefore, the nurse incorporates data obtained from skin assessment into his or her diagnostic categories.

SKIN INTEGRITY, IMPAIRED

DEFINITION
Impaired skin integrity implies a break in the skin, placing the individual at risk for a local or systemic infection.

ETIOLOGY
Physical immobility
Altered nutritional state
Medications
Chronic disease
    Diabetes mellitus
    Hepatitis
    Cirrhosis
    Renal failure
    Cancer
    Arteriosclerosis
    Anemia
    Congestive heart failure
Infections
    Bacterial
    Viral
    Fungal
Immunological deficit
Altered circulation
Radiation
Hyperthermia
Hypothermia
Trauma
Burns
Abrasions
Edema

Moisture
Skeletal prominence pressure

DEFINING CHARACTERISTICS

Regulatory Behaviors
Erythema
Red streak
Laceration
Itching
Numbness
Pain
Tenderness
Cracked skin
Excoriation
Ulceration

Cognitive Behaviors
Unknown

NURSING RESPONSIBILITIES

Assessment
Assess regulatory behaviors indicative of altered skin integrity (I)
Monitor the ECG pattern continuously (I)
Monitor the side or therapeutic effects of prescribed medications (I)
Assess the patient's prehospital skin integrity (I)
Palpate pulses for quality and equality (I)

Interventions

Fluid
Administer prescribed IV fluids (D)
Regulate the IV flow rate and check for patency (I)
Evaluate the skin for color, temperature changes, and moisture (I)
Evaluate the skin for edema (I)
Evaluate the skin for alterations in integrity: abrasions, punctures, or lacerations (I)
Evaluate laboratory studies (I)

Aeration

    Administer humidified oxygen by mask, nasal catheter, or nasal cannula at the prescribed percentage and flow rate (D)

    Evaluate the effectiveness of oxygen therapy (I)

Nutrition

    Provide a diet containing sufficient calories and proteins (I)

    Consult with the dietitian (I)

    Assist the patient with eating (I)

    Determine the patient's food preferences (I)

Communication

    Reduce the patient's anxiety level (I)

    Listen to the patient's concerns, fears, and anxieties (I)

    Arrange situations that encourage the patient's autonomy I)

    Encourage patient participation in self-care (I)

    Provide knowledge regarding the causes of alteration in skin integrity (I)

Activity

    Maintain skin integrity by keeping the skin clean and dry (I)

    Perform active and passive range-of-motion exercises (I)

    Encourage alternate rest and activity periods (I)

    Elevate an edematous extremity (I)

    Massage all bony prominences and pressure points (I)

    Change the patient's position q2h (I)

    Change dressings and/or tubings using appropriate techniques (I)

Pain

    Administer analgesics as prescribed (D)

    Evaluate the type, location, and duration of pain (I)

Bibliography

Carpenito, L. J. *Handbook of nursing diagnosis.* Philadelphia: Lippincott, 1984.

Gettrust, K., Ryan, S., & Engleman, D. *Applied nursing diagnosis.* New York: Wiley, 1985.

Gordon, M. *Manual of nursing diagnosis.* New York: McGraw-Hill, 1985.

Kelly, M. *Nursing diagnosis source book: Guidelines for clinical application.* Norwalk, Conn.: Appleton-Century-Crofts, 1985.

FLUID VOLUME DEFICIT
Actual Plasma Volume Deficit, Burn Shock

DEFINITION
Burn shock is also referred to as electrolyte shock or plasma loss shock.

ETIOLOGY
Exposure of skin to
  Fire
  High temperature of dry or moist heat
  Electricity
  x-ray
  Radium
  Corrosive chemical(s)

DEFINING CHARACTERISTICS

Regulatory Behaviors
  Pain, first- and second-degree
  Blisters
  Nausea
  Vomiting
  Hypotension
  Decreased cardiac output
  Hyperthermia
  Impaired capillary filling
  Anemia
  Fatigue
  Weakness
  Edema
  Curling's ulcer
  Oliguria
  Tachycardia
  Tachypnea

Cognitive Behaviors
  Restlessness
  Anxiety
  Discomfort
  Irritability

Confusion
Apprehension

NURSING RESPONSIBILITIES

Assessment

Assess regulatory behaviors indicative of burn shock (I)
Assess cognitive behaviors indicative of burn shock (I)
Monitor the ECG pattern continuously (I)
Observe the side or therapeutic effects of prescribed medications (I)
Inspect the skin for edema (I)
Auscultate the heart for abnormal heart sounds (I)
Palpate for arterial pulsations and peripheral pulses (I)
Auscultate the heart for rate, rhythm, and regularity (I)
Auscultate the chest for adventitious breath sounds (I)
Auscultate the chest for respiratory rate, rhythm, and regularity (I)

Interventions

Fluid

Administer prescribed medications (D)
Administer prescribed IV fluids (D)
    Plasma
    Plasma expander
    Hypertonic lactated saline (HLS)
    Electrolytes
Evaluate both degree and extent of the burns (ID)
Insert a Foley catheter (ID)
Evaluate urine for sugar and acetone (ID)
Measure the amount of fluid loss from wounds, dressings, and drainage (I)
Measure urinary volume and specific gravity (I)
Assist the physician in determining the amount of tissue loss and degree of burn (I)
Evaluate data from hemodynamic parameters: CVP, PAP, PCWP, CO, and SVR (I)
Evaluate laboratory data: BUN, potassium, hemoglobin, hematocrit, and sodium (I)
Regulate the IV flow rate (I)
Measure arterial blood pressure and MAP (I)

Aeration

> Provide oxygen at the prescribed percentage and flow rate (I)
>
> Evaluate the skin for pallor or cyanosis (I)
>
> Evaluate the breathing pattern for shortness of breath, tachypnea, or dyspnea (I)
>
> Reduce meaningless environmental stimuli (I)

Nutrition

> Administer IV hyperalimentation (D)
>
> Insert a nasogastric tube if necessary (D)

Communication

> Reduce the patient's anxiety level (I)
>
> Provide knowledge regarding diagnostic procedures and supportive devices (I)
>
> Support the family through the initial crisis (I)
>
> Inform the physician of any changes in the patient's condition (I)
>
> Listen to the patient's concerns regarding changes in his or her physical appearance (I)

Activity

> Reduce the patient's stress level so as to minimize the potential for a Curling's ulcer (I)
>
> Protect the patient against infection, since his or her immune response is reduced (I)
>
> Administer prescribed medications (D)
>
> Prepare the patient for a painful experience (I)
>
> Discuss possible pain-relieving measures (I)

Bibliography

Bordicks, K. *Patterns of shock implications for nursing care* (2nd ed.). New York: Macmillan, 1980.

Gettrust, K., Ryan, S., & Engleman, D. *Applied nursing diagnosis.* New York: Wiley, 1985.

TISSUE PERFUSION, ALTERATION IN
Vasodilatation of Vascular Bed, Septic Shock

DEFINITION

In septic shock, cardiac output is high and vascular resistance is low, thus leading to vascular collapse.

ETIOLOGY
  Gram-negative bacteria
    Escherichia coli
    Klebsiella and Aerobacter
    Pseudomonas
    Proteus
    Serratia
  Urinary tract infection
  Peritonitis
    Uterus
    Fallopian tube
    Instrumental abortion
    Intra-abdominal disease, ruptured bowel
  Hemodynamic instrumentation

DEFINING CHARACTERISTICS

Regulatory Behaviors
  Hyperdynamic phase
    Diaphoresis
    Pyrexia
    Normal to decreased urinary output
    Decreased PO_2
    Tachycardia
    Chills
    Skin flushed and warm
    Tachypnea
    Decreased systolic pressure
    Metabolic acidosis
  Normodynamic phase
    CVP normal to high
    Pulmonary congestion
    Peripheral edema
    Tachycardia
    Hypotension
    PAP normal to high
    Oliguria
    Thirst
    Progressive hypoxemia
    Hyperventilation

Hypodynamic phase
    Elevated PAP
    Profound hypoxemia
    Metabolic acidosis
    Tachycardia
    Hypotension
    Cold, clammy skin
    Tachypnea
    Elevated CVP

Cognitive Behaviors
Hyperdynamic phase
    Restlessness
    Confusion
    Irritability
Normodynamic phase
    Lassitude
    Tiredness
Hypodynamic phase
    Coma.

NURSING RESPONSIBILITIES

Assessment
Assess regulatory behaviors indicative of septic shock (I)
Assess cognitive behaviors indicative of septic shock (I)
Monitor the ECG pattern continuously (I)
Observe the side or therapeutic effects of prescribed medications (I)
Assess the patient's neurological status (I)
Inspect for peripheral edema (I)
Auscultate the heart for abnormal heart sounds (I)
Palpate for arterial pulsations and peripheral pulses (I)
Auscultate the heart for rate, rhythm, and regularity (I)
Inspect the jugular veins (I)
Palpate the chest for vocal and tactile fremitus (I)
Auscultate the chest for adventitious breath sounds (I)
Percuss the chest for abnormal resonance (I)
Auscultate the abdomen for abnormal bowel sounds (I)
Inspect the abdomen for distension (I)
Palpate the abdomen for tenderness, rigidity, and masses (I)

Interventions

Fluid

    Administer prescribed IV fluids (D)
        Ringer's lactate
        Albumisol
        Blood
    Administer prescribed medications (D)
        Dopamine
        Dobutamine
        Epinephrine
        Isuprel
        Calcium chloride
        Hydrocortisone
        Gentamicin
        Tobramycin
        Amikacin
    Evaluate blood studies for abnormal acid–base balance (I)
    Evaluate blood studies for abnormal clotting mechanisms (I)
    Evaluate serum electrolyte, BUN, and creatinine levels (I)
    Measure intake and output (I)
    Evaluate data from hemodynamic parameters: PAP, PCWP, CVP, SVR, and CO (I)

Aeration

    Administer humidified oxygen via mask, nasal catheter, or nasal prongs at the prescribed percentage and flow rate (D)
    Measure arterial blood pressure and MAP (I)
    Obtain arterial blood gasses via appropriate hemodynamic line and evaluate the results (I)
    Evaluate the skin for color, temperature, and presence of diaphoresis (I)
    Evaluate the breathing pattern for dyspnea or tachypnea (I)
    Establish and maintain a patent airway (I)
    Maintain adequate ventilation through the use of continuous ventilatory support (I)
    Suction the patient as necessary (I)
    Evaluate the effectiveness of ventilatory support, including the use of PEEP and/or weaning procedures (I)

Nutrition
    Encourage the patient to maintain a dietary intake sufficient to meet daily requirements (I)
    Consult with the dietitian (I)
    Assist the patient with eating (I)
    Incorporate the patient's food preferences, into his or her diet, when possible

Communication
    Listen to the patient's concerns, fears, and anxieties (I)
    Reduce the patient's anxiety level (I)
    Provide knowledge regarding the causes of septic shock (I)
    Encourage patient participation in self-care (I)
    Arrange situations that encourage the patient's autonomy (I)
    Support the family throughout the patient's hospitalization (I)

Activity
    Change the patient's position q2h (I)
    Encourage alternate rest and activity periods (I)
    Prevent infection by using aseptic or sterile techniques when changing tubings or dressings (I)

Pain
    Administer analgesics as prescribed (D)
    Evaluate the type, location, and duration of pain (I)
    Reduce physical discomfort that could interfere with cognitive function (I)
    Discuss possible pain-relieving measures (I)

Bibliography

Bordicks, K. *Patterns of shock implications for nursing care* (2nd ed.). New York: Macmillan, 1980.

Roberts, S. *Physiological concepts and the critically ill patient.* Englewood Cliffs, N.J.: Prentice-Hall, 1985, pp. 414–447.

POTENTIAL FOR INFECTION

DEFINITION

A clinical condition in which the individual has decreased or altered resistance to infection.

ETIOLOGY
Chronic diseases
Immunosuppressed system
Instrumentation
    Arterial line
    Swan-Ganz
Foley catheter
Trauma
Altered integumentary system
Dialysis
    Peritoneal
    Hemodialysis
Radiation therapy
Invasive procedures
Malnutrition
Medications
Prolonged immobility

DEFINING CHARACTERISTICS

Regulatory Behaviors
Local inflammation
    Redness
    Swelling
    Pain
Leukocytosis
Positive cultures
Elevated temperature
Altered immune response

Cognitive Behaviors
Unknown

NURSING RESPONSIBILITIES

Assessment
Assess regulatory behaviors indicative of infections (I)
Assess the patient's prior history with infections (I)
Observe the side or therapeutic effects of prescribed medications (I)
Inspect the skin for swelling or inflammation (I)
Auscultate the chest for adventitious breath sounds (I)

Interventions

Fluids

Administer prescribed medications (D)

Encourage fluid intake to 3000 cc/day (ID)

Evaluate all cultures and report the results to the physician (I)

Evaluate laboratory studies (I)

Measure temperature q2h or as necessary (I)

Measure arterial blood pressure and MAP (I)

Measure intake and output (I)

Aeration

Evaluate the skin for pallor or cyanosis (I)

Evaluate the breathing pattern for dyspnea, tachypnea, or shortness of breath (I)

Provide postural drainage (I)

Provide percussion and vibration (I)

Nutrition

Encourage the patient to maintain a dietary intake sufficient to meet daily requirements (I)

Consult with the dietitian (I)

Incorporate the patient's food preferences into his or her diet, when possible (I)

Communication

Limit the patient's exercise or ambulation while febrile (I)

Provide or encourage the use of diversional activities (I)

Inform the physician of elevations in the patient's temperature (I)

Inform the physician of changes in the white blood-cell count reflecting leukocytosis (I)

Instruct the patient's family in infection-control strategies (I)

Provide knowledge regarding the cause(s) of infection (I)

Activity

Provide wound care (I)

Use strict aseptic techniques during invasive procedures (I)

Provide rest between nursing interventions (I)

Prevent infection by using aseptic or sterile techniques when changing tubings or dressings (I)

Pain
   Administer prescribed analgesics (D)
   Evaluate for the presence of pain (I)
   Evaluate the location and duration of pain (I)

Bibliography

Carpenito, L. J. *Handbook of nursing diagnosis.* Philadelphia: Lippin-
   cott, 1984.
Gettrust, K., Ryan, S., & Engleman, D. *Applied nursing diagnosis.* New
   York: Wiley, 1985.

ENDOCRINE SYSTEM

The endocrine system's response to critical illness is responsi-
ble for the many biochemical and hemodynamic changes seen
in the critically ill patient. Today, patients receive hormones
(such as insulin infusion, catecholamine infusion, and steroid
boluses) as part of their treatment. Therefore, the critical care
nurse observes for physiological and emotional changes that
could indicate a hormonal imbalance. (One such imbalance is
glucose excess or deficit.)

GLUCOSE, ALTERATION IN
Serum Glucose Excess, Hyperglycemia

DEFINITION
Hyperglycemia is an acute metabolic disorder resulting from a
sustained lack of insulin.

ETIOLOGY
   Diabetic ketoacidosis
   Pancreatitis
   Salicylate intoxication
   Excess alcohol intake
   Exogenous hormone excess
   Endogenous hormone excess
   Malnutrition
   Drugs
   Infections
      Respiratory tract

Urinary tract
Skin infection
Stress
Emotional trauma
Surgery
Injury

DEFINING CHARACTERISTICS

Regulatory Behaviors
Polydipsia
Polyuria
Polyphagia
Anorexia
Nausea
Vomiting
Weakness
Malaise
Abdominal pain and tenderness
Abdominal distension
Hepatomegaly
Headache
Flushed skin
Dry skin
Tachycardia
Hyperthermia
Hypothermia
Kussmaul's respiration
Thirst
Decrease in or absence of reflexes

Cognitive Behaviors
Lethargy
Drowsiness
Confusion
Coma

NURSING RESPONSIBILITIES

Assessment
Assess regulatory behaviors indicative of hyperglycemia (I)
Assess cognitive behaviors indicative of hyperglycemia (I)

Monitor the ECG pattern continuously (I)

Observe the side or therapeutic effects of prescribed medications (I)

Assess the patient's neurological status: pupillary reactions, sensory/motor changes, level of consciousness, and vital signs (I)

Auscultate the heart for abnormal heart sounds (I)

Auscultate the heart for rate, rhythm, and regularity (I)

Inspect the jugular veins (I)

Inspect the skin for edema (I)

Inspect the skin for dehydration (I)

Auscultate the chest for adventitious breath sounds (I)

Auscultate the chest for respiratory rate, rhythm, and regularity (I)

Palpate the pulses for quality and bilateral equality (I)

Inspect for Kussmaul's respiration (I)

Inspect for cyanosis (I)

Palpate for vocal or tactile fremitus (I)

Percuss the chest for abnormal resonance (I)

Auscultate the abdomen for abnormal bowel sounds (I)

Inspect the abdomen for distension (I)

Palpate the abdomen for tenderness, rigidity, and masses (I)

Interventions

Fluid

Administer prescribed IV fluids (D)
  Isotonic saline (0.9%)
      500–1000 mL/h for 2–3 h
  Ringer's lactate
  5% D/0.45 saline
      250 mL/h

Administer prescribed medications (D)
  High-dose insulin therapy
  Low-dose insulin therapy

Replace electrolytes: sodium, potassium, phosphorus, and bicarbonate (D)

Evaluate the skin for color, temperature, and presence of diaphoresis (I)

Measure arterial blood pressure and MAP (I)

Evaluate data from hemodynamic parameters: PAP, PCWP, CVP, SVR, and CO (I)

Measure oral, nasogastric, and parenteral intake (I)

Measure urinary volume, nasogastric output, and specific gravity (I)

Regulate the IV flow rate and check for patency (I)

Evaluate laboratory studies: serum electrolytes, ketones, BUN, lipid levels, blood glucose, WBC, and hematocrit (I)

Evaluate urine sugar and acetone (I)

Weigh the patient daily (I)

Aeration

Administer humidified oxygen by mask, nasal catheter, or nasal prongs at the prescribed percentage and flow rate (D)

Evaluate arterial blood gasses (I)

Evaluate with the physician the patient's chest film (I)

Maintain a patent airway (I)

Maintain adequate ventilation through the use of continuous ventilatory support (I)

Suction the patient via airway, endotracheal tube, or tracheostomy as needed (I)

Nutrition

Provide the prescribed diet of carbohydrates and calories (D)

Administer prescribed nasogastric tube feedings (ID)

Measure drainage from the nasogastric tube (I)

Review the patient's dietary intake with him or her to determine adherence to the prescribed diet (I)

Reduce meaningless environmental stimuli (I)

Provide a spiritual support system (I)

Communication

Reduce the patient's anxiety level (I)

Reduce the family's anxiety level (I)

Provide knowledge regarding the causes and treatment of hyperglycemia (I)

Explain anticipated procedures involved in the diagnostic process (I)

Encourage decision making (I)

Encourage patient self-performance (I)

Inform the patient what is expected of him or her in critical care (I)

Arrange situations that encourage the patient's autonomy (I)

Activity

Apply appropriate antiseptic around the IV tubing connections to prevent infection (I)

Change the patient's position q2h (I)

Elevate the edematous extremity (I)

Encourage alternative rest and activity periods (I)

Reduce the demand for cognitive functioning when the patient is ill or fatigued (I)

Pain

Administer prescribed analgesics (D)

Ask the patient what makes him or her comfortable (I)

Evaluate the type, location, and duration of pain (I)

Bibliography

Johanson, B., Dungca, C., Hoffmeister, D., & Wells, S. *Standards for critical care* (2nd ed.). St. Louis: C. V. Mosby, 1985.

Roberts, S. *Physiological concepts and the critically ill patient.* Englewood Cliffs, N.J.: Prentice-Hall, 1985, pp. 310–339.

Serum Glucose Deficit, Hypoglycemia

DEFINITION

Hypoglycemia is a metabolic disorder resulting from an increase in insulin and a decrease in glucose levels < 50 mg/dL.

ETIOLOGY

Reactive hypoglycemia (exogenous causes)

Functional idiopathy

Fructose, galactose, amino acid intolerance

Postgastrectomy

Drugs

Insulin

Sulfonylurea

Alcohol

Fasting hypoglycemia (endogenous processes)

Alcohol

Insulin therapy

Pancreatic disease

Extensive liver disease

Insulinoma

Neoplastic disease
Adrenoenteral insufficiency
Congestive heart failure
Starvation
Exercise
Oral hypoglycemic agents
Pregnancy
Fever

DEFINING CHARACTERISTICS

Regulatory Behaviors
Headache
Weakness
Tremors
Palpitations
Nausea
Blurred vision
Pallor
Diaphoresis
Tachycardia
Increased systolic pressure
Dilated pupils
Seizure

Cognitive Behaviors
Nervousness
Anxiety
Confusion
Depression
Lethargy
Bizarre behavior
Stupor

NURSING RESPONSIBILITIES

Assessment
Assess regulatory behaviors indicative of hypoglycemia (I)
Assess cognitive behaviors indicative of hypoglycemia (I)
Monitor the ECG pattern continuously (I)
Observe the side or therapeutic effects of prescribed medications (I)

Assess neurological status: pupillary reaction, sensory/motor changes, level of consciousness, and vital signs (I)

Inspect for pallor (I)

Auscultate the chest for respiratory rate, rhythm, and regularity (I)

Inspect the eyes for pupil size, equality, and response to light (I)

Interventions

Fluids

Administer 50 ml of 50% glucose IV for the unconscious patient (D)

Administer epinephrine or glucagon (D)

Evaluate serum-glucose levels (I)

Evaluate the skin for color, temperature, and presence of diaphoresis (I)

Measure arterial blood pressure and MAP (I)

Measure intake, urinary volume, and specific gravity (I)

Evaluate laboratory studies (I)

Evaluate the patient's urine for sugar and acetone (I)

Aeration

Evaluate the breathing pattern for shortness of breath or dyspnea (I)

Nutrition

Provide sweetened orange juice or tea with honey (I)

Instruct the patient to restrict the use of simple sugars (I)

Instruct the patient to eat small, frequent meals (I)

Restrict the use of beverages containing caffeine (I)

Consult with the dietitian (I)

Communication

Provide knowledge regarding the causes of hypoglycemia (I)

Encourage patient self-performance (I)

Reduce the patient's anxiety level (I)

Arrange situations that encourage the patient's autonomy (I)

Activity

Evaluate for tremors and weakness before encouraging unsupervised ambulation (I)

Reduce the demands for cognitive functioning when the patient is ill or fatigued (I)

Evaluate any alterations in the patient's thought process (I)

Protect the patient during seizure activity (I)

Encourage rest periods following nursing interventions (I)

Pain

Administer prescribed medications (D)

Evaluate for the presence of pain (I)

Ask the patient what makes him or her comfortable (I)

Bibliography

Borg, N., Nikas, D., Stark, J., & Williams, S. *Core curriculum for critical care nursing.* Philadelphia: W. B. Saunders, 1981.

Johanson, B., Dungca, C., Hoffmeister, D., & Wells S. *Standards for critical care* (2nd ed.). St. Louis: C. V. Mosby, 1985.

7

Major Diagnostic Categories and Nursing Diagnostic Categories

Health care costs in the United States have been steadily rising to astronomical levels over the past decade. In addition, the mean age of our population has also been rising. Therefore, more people 65 years of age and older will eventually require some form of medical care. Since 1966, the federal government, through Medicare, has been the chief financier of health care to the elderly. With the rising cost of health care, the expansion of existing programs (due to the development of sophisticated technology), and the steadily increasing number of Medicare clients, the federal government has been considering ways to contain or reduce costs.

As a result of a study conducted by Yale University, the prospective reimbursement system of payment was created. The researchers at Yale created the Diagnostic Related Groups (DRGs) system. It is based upon the International Classification of Diseases drawn up by the World Health Organization in the 1920s.

MAJOR DIAGNOSTIC CATEGORIES

In 1982, President Reagan signed Public Law 98–21, the Social Security Amendment of 1983. Title VI of this law changes the way in which Medicare determines how much hospitals are reimbursed for inpatient care. The prospective payment system, based upon DRGs, brings clinical and financial data together (Shaffer, 1984).

In 1983, the prospective reimbursement system was implemented. Prospective reimbursement is defined as a "cost containment strategy wherein an external authority establishes the prices that providers are allowed to charge and/or that third parties are required to pay for specified services in advance of the period in which the services are actually provided" (Dowling, 1976, pp. 7–37). According to Linammod, "prospective reimbursement is to be budget neutral: the law requires that Medicare reimbursement not exceed amounts that would have been paid under cost-based reimbursement" (1985, p. 96).

DRGs were developed according to specific factors regarding reimbursement. The factors consist of medical diagnosis, complications, age, and surgical procedures utilized. Each DRG has a predetermined dollar price that is based upon an average cost per case in that category. Therefore, Medicare payments are made according to a predetermined rate for each discharge. The payment is based upon a diagnosis made from the 468 DRGs.

It is the hope of the federal government that the system of prospective reimbursement will save them $13 million or more a year. Should a patient be discharged before the allotted time, the hospital gets to keep the difference between the actual cost of caring for the patient and the amount of money paid by the government. Likewise, should a patient remain hospitalized beyond the allotted time, the hospital loses money. Therein lies the motivation to provide the best care possible while moving the patient along so that he or she is discharged within the allotted time (Smith, 1985).

The prospective reimbursement system has implications for nursing. According to Wake and colleagues, "given current trends in reimbursement, the development of a diagnostic classification system will surely impact on the type of staffing and quality of care available to patients in critical care units of the future" (1985, pp. 447–448). While hospitals use DRGs to both categorize patient care and receive payment, in the near future, nurses may be called upon to further develop their own reimbursement system. One way to accomplish this goal is through the use of Nursing Diagnostic Related Groups (NDRGs).

NURSING DIAGNOSTIC CATEGORIES

According to Wake and colleagues: "Critical care nurses have a vantage point and a perspective about nursing practice that differs from nurses providing care in other settings. Their expressed concern about nursing diagnostic categories, especially the absence of phenomena for which they purport to assume responsibility and accountability, must be viewed as legitimate and could provide the bases for verbal and written dialogue across widely separated specialty boundaries" (1985, p. 447).

Nurses are using nursing diagnoses with increasing frequency as they plan and implement their nursing care. Traditionally, nursing diagnoses have been labels created by nurses for those conditions that are correlated with their knowledge and their legal treatment domain. Today, nurses have tremendous expertise in making assessments and in making a wide range of both physiological and psychosocial nursing diagnoses. Their nursing diagnoses are based upon an ever-expanding body of scientific knowledge. This is especially true in critical care, where technology, scientific knowledge, and nursing responsibilities have simultaneously expanded.

Critical care nurses can increase their skill and knowledge in diagnostic judgment with continued practice in diagnostic thinking. Like physicians, nurses collect data regarding the patient's potential or actual health problems; analyze the data by isolating significant findings, cluster related facts, attach meaning to the clusters and, finally, state a nursing diagnosis (Kelly, 1985).

Major diagnostic categories, including DRGs, are here to stay. They may be modified in the near future based upon how hospitals view their success or failure. Nevertheless, the concept of prospective reimbursement as a cost-saving strategy will remain. Therefore, nurses can use the newness of the reimbursement system to their own advantage. Critical care nurses involved in clinical practice use both medical-focussed and nursing-focussed diagnostic thinking. Hence, it seems natural that the DRG and NDRG classifications should be jointly used.

Nurses can use Nursing Diagnostic Categories or Nursing Diagnostic Related Groups to establish a code of repayment for their care. A patient can be charged for a particular nursing diagnosis, cluster of nursing diagnoses, or interventions for each nursing diagnosis. To this end, nurses need to refine existing nursing diagnoses and to develop a wider range, or more specific, behavioral/psychosocial and physiological nursing diagnoses.

NDRGs may become imperative for critical care nurses who are concerned with supporting the need for 2:1 versus 4:1 patient-nurse ratios. Some believe that outsiders may view critical care staffing, with its 2:1 patient-nurse ratio, as an area in which to streamline a hospital's budget. Some may argue that an increase in the number of patients might actually increase the average length of stay (LOS), thereby increasing the cost of the average hospital stay (Erickson, 1985). Therefore, it is important that critical care nurses develop collaborative nursing diagnoses to the advantage of both nurses and the patients' well-being.

Nurses, including critical care nurses, can use NDRGs to provide patient care and to facilitate continuity of care. For example, a critical care nurse may diagnose a knowledge deficit related to the causes, treatment, and prognosis of myocardial infarction. Interventions can be developed for the patient's entire hospitalization. In this respect, the critical care nurse and the intermediate or step-down nurse can provide continuity of care by following the patient's progress with the diagnosis of "knowledge deficit." Both units can benefit from the combined reimbursement.

This chapter lists DRGs as they fall into a particular major diagnostic category. For each major diagnostic category, a list of potential behavioral and/or collaborative nursing diagnoses has been provided. The nursing diagnoses are simply listed and are not in any particular order. Therefore, while they appear opposite a particular DRG, the two are not correlated. The following is an example of a DRG and possible nursing diagnoses (Grimaldi and Micheletti, 1983).

DISEASES AND DISORDERS OF THE NERVOUS SYSTEM

Major Diagnostic Category DRG	Nursing Diagnostic Categories NDRG
10 M Nervous system neoplasms age > 69 and/or Dx 2	Thought process altered; confusion Verbal/nonverbal communication deficit Impaired physical mobility, hemiparesis Activity intolerance Hopelessness Denial Body-image changes Depression Intracranial pressure increased Central nervous system altered, seizure Speech pattern altered, aphasia

The NDRGs given above can occur at any time during the patient's hospitalization. The critical care nurse chooses the nursing diagnoses that are appropriate for the patient, depending upon the specific DRG, severity of illness, or phase of hospitalization.

DISEASES AND DISORDERS OF THE NERVOUS SYSTEM

Major Diagnostic Categories DRG	Nursing Diagnostic Categories NDRG
1 S Craniotomy age > 17 except for trauma 2 S Craniotomy for trauma age > 17	Thought process altered, confusion Verbal/nonverbal communication deficit

3 S Craniotomy age < 18	Diversional activity deficit
4 S Spinal procedures	Role disturbance
5 S Extracranial vascular procedures	Sexual dysfunction
6 S Carpal tunnel release	Impaired physical mobility, hemiparesis
7 S Peripheral + cranial nerve + other nervous system procedures age > 69 and/or diagnosis (DX) 2	Impaired physical mobility, hemiplegia Activity intolerance
8 S Peripheral + cranial nerve + other nervous system procedures < 70 without DX 2	Hopelessness Depersonalization
9 M Spinal disorders + injuries	Powerlessness
10 M Nervous system neoplasms age > 69 and/or DX 2	Denial Anger
11 M Nervous system neoplasms age < 70 without DX 2	Body image disturbance Anxiety
12 M Degenerative nervous system disorder	Fear
13 M Multiple sclerosis + cerebral ataxia	Depression
14 M Specific cerebrovascular disorders except transient ischemic attacks (TIA)	Pain Stress
15 M TIA	Sensory deprivation
16 M Nonspecific cerebrovascular disorders with DX 2	Carbon dioxide gas exchange impaired, hypercapnia
17 M Nonspecific cerebrovascular disorders without DX 2	Acid–base imbalance, respiratory acidosis
18 M Cranial + peripheral nerve disorders age > 69 and/or DX 2	Ineffective breathing pattern, dyspnea Oxygen–carbon dioxide gas exchange imbalance, crackles

19 M Cranial + peripheral nerve disorders age < 70 without DX 2 — Urinary output increased, polyuria

Oral mucous membrane, alteration in

20 M Nervous system infection, except viral meningitis — Skin integrity impaired

Potential for infection

21 M Viral meningitis — Intracranial pressure increased

22 M Hypertensive encephalopathy — Central nervous system (CNS) altered, seizure

23 M Nontraumatic stupor + coma — Extracellular fluid volume excess, cerebral edema

24 M Seizure + headache age > 69 and/or DX 2

25 M Seizure + headache age 18–69 without DX 2 — Thought process altered, loss of consciousness

26 M Seizure + headache age 0–17

27 M Traumatic stupor + coma, coma > 1 hr — Cerebral tissue perfusion, decreased

28 M Traumatic stupor + coma, coma < 1 hr age > 69 and/or DX 2 — Knowledge deficit

Cerebral perfusion obstructed, thromboembolism

29 M Traumatic stupor + coma < 1 hr age 18–69 without DX 2 — Speech pattern altered, aphasia

30 M Traumatic stupor + coma < 1 hr age 0–17 — Vasodilation of vascular bed, neurogenic shock

31 M Concussion age > 69 and/or DX 2 — Injury, limb trauma

32 M Concussion age 19–69 without DX 2 — Self-care deficit

33 M Concussion age 0–17

34 M Other disorders of nervous system age > 69 and/or DX 2

35 M Other disorders of nervous system age < 70 without DX 2

DISEASES AND DISORDERS OF THE EYE

Major Diagnostic Categories DRG	Nursing Diagnostic Categories NDRG
36 S Retinal procedures	Thought process altered, confusion
37 S Orbital procedures	Diversional activity deficit
38 S Primary iris procedures	Loneliness
39 S Lens procedures	Powerlessness
40 S Extraocular procedures except orbit age > 17	Anger
	Denial
41 S Extraocular procedures except orbit age 0–17	Self-concept/self-esteem disturbance
	Body image disturbance
42 S Intraocular procedures except retina, iris + lens	Anxiety
	Fear
43 M Hyphema	Loss
44 M Acute major eye infections	Pain
45 M Neurological eye disorders	Sensory deprivation
46 M Other disorders of the eye age > 17 with DX 2	Bowel elimination decreased, constipation
47 M Other disorders of the eye age > 17 without DX 2	Potential for infection
	Self-care deficit
48 M Other disorders of the eye age 0–17	Health maintenance altered

DISEASES AND DISORDERS OF THE EAR, NOSE, AND THROAT

Major Diagnostic Categories DRG	Nursing Diagnostic Categories NDRG
49 S Major head + neck procedures	Verbal/nonverbal communication deficit
50 S Sialoadenectomy	Diversional activity deficit

51 S Salivary gland procedures except sialodenectomy

Role disturbance
Sexual dysfunction

52 S Cleft lip + palate repair

Activity intolerance

53 S Sinus + mastoid procedures age > 17

Powerlessness

54 S Sinus + mastoid procedures age 0–17

Denial

55 S Miscellaneous ear, nose + throat procedures

Anger

56 S Rhinoplasty

Body image

57 S Tonsillectomy + Adenoidectomy procedures except tonsillectomy and/or adenoidectomy age > 17

Anxiety
Fear

58 S Tonsillectomy + Adenoidectomy procedures except tonsillectomy and/or adenoidectomy age 0–17

Depression
Loss

59 S Tonsillectomy and/or adenoidectomy age > 17

Pain
Sensory deprivation

60 S Tonsillectomy and/or adenoidectomy age 0–17

Sleep deprivation
Bowel elimination decreased, constipation

61 S Myringotomy age > 17

Nutritional alteration, less than body requirements

62 S Myringotomy age 0–17

63 S Other ear, nose + throat O.R. procedures

64 M Ear, nose + throat malignancy

Knowledge deficit

65 M Disequilibrium

Ineffective airway clearance, obstruction

66 M Epistaxis

67 M Epiglottis

Health maintenance, altered

68 M Otitis media + upper respiratory infections (URI) > 69 and/or DX 2

Oral mucous membrane, altered

69 M Otitis media + URI age 18–69 without DX 2

Swallowing pattern, altered, facial trauma

70 M Otitis media + URI age 0–17

71 M Laryngotracheitis   Potential for infection
72 M Nasal trauma + defor-   Self-care deficit
    mity
73 M Other ear, nose + throat
    diagnoses age > 17
74 M Other ear, nose + throat
    diagnoses age 0–17

DISEASES AND DISORDERS OF THE RESPIRATORY SYSTEM

Major Diagnostic Categories DRG	Nursing Diagnostic Categories NDRG
75 S Major chest procedures	Thought process altered, confusion
76 S O.R. procedures on the respiratory system except major chest with DX 2	Verbal/nonverbal communication deficit
	Verbal/nonverbal communication excess
77 S O.R. procedures on the respiratory system except major chest without DX 2	Violence directed toward others
78 M Pulmonary embolism	Noncompliance
79 M Respiratory infection + inflammations age > 69 and/or DX 2	Diversional activity deficit
	Role disturbance
	Sexual dysfunction
80 M Respiratory infections + inflammation age 18–69 without DX 2	Knowledge deficit
	Psychological immobility
81 M Respiratory infections + inflammations age 0–17	Activity intolerance
	Hopelessness
82 M Respiratory neoplasms	Powerlessness
83 M Major chest trauma age > 69 and/or DX 2	Anger
84 M Major chest trauma age > 70 without DX 2	Body image disturbance
85 M Pleural effusion age > 69 and/or DX 2	Anxiety

86 M Pleural effusion age < 70 without DX 2	Fear
87 M Pulmonary edema + respiratory failure	Depression
88 M Chronic obstructive pulmonary disease	Loss
89 M Simple pneumonia + pleurisy age > 69 and/or DX 2	Pain Sensory deprivation
90 M Simple pneumonia + pleurisy age 18–69 without DX 2	Sensory overload Stress
91 M Simple pneumonia + pleurisy age 0–17	Sleep deprivation
92 M Interstitial lung disease age > 69 and/or DX 2	Alteration in right ventricular-atrial preload
93 M Interstitial lung disease age < 70 without DX 2	Alteration in left ventricular-atrial preload
94 M Pneumothorax age > 69 and/or DX 2	Alteration in cardiopulmonary stability, chest injury shock
95 M Pneumothorax age < 70 without DX 2	
96 M Bronchitis + asthma age > 69 and/or DX 2	Cardiac output decreased
97 M Bronchitis + asthma age 18–69 without DX 2	Extracellular fluid volume excess, alveolar edema
98 M Bronchitis + asthma age 0–17	
99 M Respiratory signs + symptoms age > 69 and/or DX 2	Oxygen gas exchange impaired, hypoxemia
100 M Respiratory signs + symptoms age < 70 without DX 2	Carbon dioxide gas exchange impaired, hypercapnia
101 M Other respiratory age > 69 and/or DX 2	Acid–base imbalance, respiratory acidosis
102 M Other respiratory diagnoses age < 70 without DX 2	Acid–base imbalance, respiratory alkalosis Ineffective breathing pattern, alveolar hypoventilation

Ineffective breathing pattern, alveolar hyperventilation

Ineffective breathing pattern, dyspnea

Oxygen–carbon dioxide gas exchange impaired, crackles

Ineffective airway clearance, wheezes

Alteration in pulmonary tissue perfusion, emboli

Alteration in distributive gas exchange, spontaneous pneumothorax

Ventilation–perfusion imbalance

Extracellular fluid volume excess, edema

Acid–base imbalance, metabolic acidosis

Aicd–base imbalance, metabolic alkalosis

Nutritional alteration, less than body requirements

Oral mucous membrane, alteration

Skin integrity impaired

Potential for infection

Injury, chest trauma

Self-care deficit

DISEASES AND DISORDERS OF THE CIRCULATORY SYSTEM

Major Diagnostic Categories DRG	Nursing Diagnostic Categories NDRG
103 S Heart transplant	Thought process altered, confusion
104 S Combined with 105	Noncompliance

105 S Cardiac valve procedure with pump (with and without catheterization)

Role disturbance
Sexual dysfunction

106 S Combined with 107

107 S Coronary bypass (with and without catheterization

Knowledge deficit
Health maintenance, altered
Impaired physical mobility, weakness

108 S Cardiothoracic procedures except valve + coronary bypass, with pump

Psychological immobility
Activity intolerance

109 S Cardiothoracic procedures without pump

110 S Major reconstructive vascular procedures age > 69 and/or DX 2

Hopelessness
Powerlessness
Depersonalization
Anger

111 S Major reconstructive vascular procedures age < 70 without DX 2

Denial
Anxiety

112 S Vascular procedures except major reconstruction

Fear
Depression

113 S Amputation for circulatory system disorders except upper limb + toe

Loss
Pain

114 S Upper limb + toes amputation for circulatory system disorders

Stress
Sensory overload

115 S Permanent cardiac pacemaker implant with AMI or congestive heart failure (CHF)

Sleep deprivation
Alteration in right ventricular–atrial preload

116 S Permanent cardiac pacemaker implant without AMI or CHF

Alteration in left ventricular–atrial preload

117 S Cardiac pacemaker replace + revision except pulse generator replacement only

Alteration in systemic vascular resistance, afterload

118 S Cardiac pacemaker pulse generator replacement only	Cardiac output decreased
119 S Vein ligation + stripping	Cardiac output increased
120 S Other O.R. procedures on the circulatory system	Arterial blood pressure altered, hypotension
121 M Combined with 122	Arterial blood pressure altered, hypertension
122 M Circulatory disorders with AMI with and without complications discharge cardiovascular alive	Coronary artery perfusion decreased
123 M Circulatory disorders with AMI, expired	Peripheral tissue perfusion decreased
124 M Circulatory disorders except AMI with catheter complicated CX 1	Peripheral tissue perfusion obstructed, thrombophlebitis
125 M Circulatory disorders except AMI, with cardiac catheter uncomplicated DX 1	Cardiopulmonary stability altered, chest injury shock
126 M Acute + subacute endocarditis	Actual reduction in cardiac output, cardiogenic shock
127 M Heart failure + shock	
128 M Deep vein thrombosis	Vasodilatation of vascular bed, anaphylactic shock
129 M Cardiac arrest	
130 M Peripheral vascular disorders age > 69 and/or DX 2	Sinus conduction alteration, sinus arrhythmia
131 M Peripheral vascular disorders age < 70 without DX 2	Sinus conduction, alteration, sinus tachycardia
132 M Atherosclerosis age > 69 and/or DX 2	Sinus conduction alteration, sinus bradycardia
133 M Atherosclerosis age < 70 without DX 2	
134 M Hypertension	Sinus conduction alteration, sinus pause or block
135 M Cardiac congenital + valvular disorders age > 69 and/or DX 2	

136 M Cardiac congenital +
valvular disorders age
18–69 without DX 2

137 M Cardiac congenital +
valvular disorders age 0–17

138 M Cardiac arrhythmia +
conduction disorders age
> 69 and/or DX 2

139 M Cardiac arrhythmia +
conduction disorders age
< 70 without DX 2

140 M Angina pectoris

141 M Syncope + collapse age
> 69 and/or DX 2

142 M Syncope + collapse age
< 70 without DX 2

143 M Chest pain

144 M Other circulatory diagnoses with DX 2

145 M Other circulatory diagnoses without DX 2

Sinus conduction alteration,
sinoatrial (SA) exit block

Atrial conduction alteration,
premature atrial contrac-
tion

Atrial conduction alteration,
paroxysmal atrial tachy-
cardia

Atrial conduction alteration,
atrial flutter

Atrial conduction alteration,
atrial fibrillation

Atrio–ventricular conduction
alteration, junctional
tachycardia

Atrio–ventricular conduction
alteration, premature junctional systole

Atrio–ventricular conduction
alteration, first-degree block

Atrio-ventricular conduction
alteration, Mobitz Type I

Atrio–ventricular conduction
alteration, Mobitz Type II

Atrio–ventricular conduction
alteration, complete heart
block

Ventricular conduction alteration, premature ventricular
beat

Ventricular conduction alteration, ventricular tachy-
cardia

Ventricular conduction alteration, ventricular fibrillation

Ventricular conduction alteration, accelerated idioventricular rhythm

Extracellular fluid volume
excess, alveolar edema

Oxygen gas exchange impaired, hypoxemia

Oxygen gas exchange impaired, hypercapnia

Carbon dioxide gas exchange impaired, respiratory acidosis

Carbon dioxide gas exchange impaired, respiratory alkalosis

Ineffective breathing pattern, dyspnea

Oxygen–carbon dioxide gas exchange impaired, crackles

Ineffective airway clearance, wheezes

Ventilation–perfusion imbalance

Extracellular fluid-volume excess, edema

Intracellular electrolyte deficit, hypokalemia

Urinary output decreased, oliguria

Potential for infection

Self-care deficit

DISEASES AND DISORDERS OF THE DIGESTIVE SYSTEM

Major Diagnostic Categories DRG	Nursing Diagnostic Categories NDRG
146 S Rectal resection age > 69 and/or DX 2	Noncompliance
147 S Rectal resection age < 70 without DX 2	Diversional activity deficit
	Role disturbance

148 S Major small + large
bowel procedures age > 69
and/or DX 2

Sexual dysfunction
Psychological immobility

149 S Major small + large
bowel procedures age < 70
without DX 2

Activity intolerance
Impaired physical mobility,
weakness

150 S Peritoneal adhesiolysis
age > 69 and/or DX 2

Powerlessness
Anger

151 S Peritoneal adhesiolysis
age < 70 without DX 2

Denial
Body image disturbance

152 S Minor small + large
bowel procedures age > 69
and/or DX 2

Anxiety
Fear

153 S Minor small + large
bowel procedures age < 70
without DX 2

Depression
Pain

154 S Stomach, esophageal +
duodenal procedures age
> 69 and/or DX 2

Loss
Extracellular fluid-volume
excess alveolar edema

155 S Stomach, esophageal +
duodenal procedures age
18–69 without DX 2

Ineffective breathing pattern,
alveolar hypoventilation

156 S Stomach, esophageal +
duodenal procedures age
0–17

Carbon dioxide gas exchange
impaired, respiratory
acidosis

157 S Anal procedures age
> 69 and/or DX 2

158 S Anal procedures age
< 70 without DX 2

Extracellular fluid-volume
excess, edema

159 S Hernia procedures
except inguinal + femoral
age > 69 and/or DX 2

Intracellular electrolyte excess, hyperkalemia

160 S Hernia procedures
except inguinal + femoral
age 18–69 without DX 2

Intracellular electrolyte deficit, hypokalemia

161 S Inguinal + femoral
hernia procedures age
> 69 and/or DX 2

Extracellular electrolyte
excess, hypernatremia

162 S Inguinal + femoral
hernia procedures age
18–69 without DX 2

Extracellular electrolyte
deficit, hyponatremia

163 S Hernia procedures age 0–17 — Intracellular electrolyte excess, hypermagnesium

164 S Appendectomy with complicated principle diagnosis age > 69 and/or DX 2 — Intracellular electrolyte deficit, hypomagnesium

165 S Appendectomy with complicated principle diagnosis age < 70 without DX 2 — Urinary output, decreased, oliguria

166 S Appendectomy without complicated principle diagnosis age > 69 and/or DX 2 — Knowledge deficit
Bowel elimination decreased, constipation

167 S Appendectomy without complicated principle diagnosis age < 70 without DX 2 — Bowel elimination increased, diarrhea

168 S Procedures on the mouth age > 69 and/or DX 2 — Bowel elimination uncontrolled, incontinence

169 S Procedures on the mouth age < 70 without DX 2 — Extracellular fluid volume excess, intraperitoneal edema or ascites

170 S Other digestive system procedures age > 69 and/or DX 2 — Decreased intraabdominal perfusion

171 S Other digestive system procedures age < 70 without DX 2 — Nutritional alteration, less than body requirements

172 M Digestive malignancy age > 69 and/or DX 2 — Nutritional alteration, more than body requirements

173 M Digestive malignancy age < 70 without DX 2 — Swallowing pattern altered, dysphagia

174 M Gastrointestinal hemorrhage age > 69 and/or DX 2 — Oral mucous membrane, alteration in

175 M Gastrointestinal hemorrhage age < 70 without DX 2 — Skin integrity, impaired
Potential for infection

176 M Complicated peptic

177 M Uncomplicated peptic ulcer > 69 and/or DX 2

178 M Uncomplicated peptic ulcer < 70 without DX 2

179 M Inflammatory bowel disease

180 M Gastrointestinal obstruction age > 69 and/or DX 2

181 M Gastrointestinal obstruction age < 70 without DX 2

182 M Esophagitis, gastroenteritis + miscellaneous digestive disorders age > 69 and/or DX 2

183 M Esophagitis, gastroenteritis + digestive disorders age 18–69 without DX 2

184 M Esophagitis, gastroenteritis + miscellaneous digestive disorders age 0–17

185 M Dental + oral disorders except extractions + restorations, age > 17

186 M Dental + oral disorders except extractions + restorations, age 0–17

187 M Dental extractions + restorations

188 M Other digestive system diagnoses age > 69 and/or DX 2

189 M Other digestive system diagnoses age 18–69 without DX 2

190 M Other digestive system diagnoses age 0–17

Self-care deficit

Injury, blunt abdominal trauma

Injury, penetrating abdominal trauma

DISEASES AND DISORDERS OF THE HEPATOBILIARY SYSTEM AND PANCREAS

Major Diagnostic Categories DRG	Nursing Diagnostic Categories NDRG
191 S Major pancreas, liver + shunt procedures	Thought process altered, confusion
192 S Minor pancreas, liver + shunt procedures	Violence directed toward self
193 S Biliary tract procedures except total cholecystectomy age > 69 and/or DX 2	Violence directed toward others
194 S Biliary tract procedures except total cholecystectomy age < 70 without DX 2	Diversional activity deficit
	Role disturbance
	Knowledge deficit
195 S Combined with 197	Impaired physical mobility, muscle weakness
196 S Combined with 198	Impaired physical mobility, shortness of breath
197 S Total cholecystectomy with and without common duct exploration age > 69 and/or DX 2	
198 S Total cholecystectomy with and without common diagnostic exploration age < 70 without DX 2	Hopelessness
	Powerlessness
199 S Hepatobiliary diagnostic procedures for malignancy	Anger
200 S Hepatobiliary diagnostic procedures for non-malignancy	Denial
	Self-concept/self-esteem disturbance
201 S Other hepatobiliary or pancreas O.R. procedures	Body image disturbance
	Anxiety
202 M Cirrhosis + alcoholic hepatitis	Fear
203 M Malignancy of hepatobiliary system or pancreas	Depression
	Pain

204 M Disorders of pancreas
except malignancy

205 M Disorders of liver
except malignant cirrhosis
+ alcoholic hepatitis age
> 69 and/or DX 2

206 M Disorders of liver
except malignant cirrhosis
+ alcoholic hepatitis age
< 70 without DX 2

207 M Disorders of the biliary
tract age > 69 and/or DX 2

208 M Disorders of the biliary
tract age < 70 without
DX 2

Knowledge deficit

Sensory deprivation
Sleep deprivation

Stress
Alteration in right ventricular-
atrial preload

Alteration in left ventricular-
atrial preload
Alteration in systemic vascular
resistance, afterload
Cardiac output decreased
Arterial blood pressure
altered, hypotension
Oxygen gas exchange im-
paired, hypoxemia
Ineffective breathing pattern,
alveolar hyperventilation
Ineffective breathing pattern,
dyspnea
Oxygen–carbon dioxide gas
exchange impaired, crackles
Extracellular fluid volume
excess, edema
Actual whole blood volume
deficit, hemorrhagic shock
Urinary output decreased,
oliguria
Actual fluid volume and electrolyte deficit, diabetic
shock
Acid–base imbalance, metabolic acidosis
Extracellular fluid volume
excess, intraperitoneal
edema or ascites

Nutritional alteration, less
than body requirements
Oral mucous membrane,
alteration in
Skin integrity impaired
Self-care deficit
Serum glucose excess, hyper-
glycemia
Serum glucose deficit, hypo-
glycemia

DISEASES OF THE MUSCULOSKELETAL SYSTEM AND CONNECTIVE TISSUE

Major Diagnostic Categories DRG	Nursing Diagnostic Categories NDRG
210 S Hip + femur procedures except major joint age > 69 and/or DX 2	Diversional activity deficit Role disturbance
211 S Hip + femur procedures except major joint age 18–69 without DX 2	Sexual dysfunction Impaired physical mobility, muscular weakness
212 S Hip + femur procedures except major joint age 0–17	Impaired physical mobility, hemiparesis
213 S Amputations for musculoskeletal system + connective tissue disorders	Activity intolerance Knowledge deficit
214 S Back + neck procedures age > 69 and/or DX 2	Loneliness Hopelessness
215 S Back + neck procedures age < 70 without DX 2	Depersonalization
216 S Biopsies of musculoskeletal system + connective tissue	Powerlessness Anger
217 S Wound debridement + skin graft except hand, for musculoskeletal + connective tissue disorders	Denial Body image disturbance

218 S Lower extremity +
humerus procedures except
hip, foot, femur age > 69
and/or DX 2

Anxiety
Fear

219 S Lower extremity +
humerus procedures except
hip, foot, femur age 18–69
without DX 2

Loss
Pain

220 S Lower extremity +
humerus procedures except
hip, foot, femur age 0–17

Sensory deprivation
Sleep deprivation

221 S Knee procedures age
> 69 and/or DX 2

Obstructed peripheral tissue
perfusion, thrombophle-
bitis

222 S Knee procedures age
< 70 without DX 2

223 S Upper extremity procedures except humerus +
hand age > 69 and/or
DX 2

Skin integrity impaired
Vasodilatation of vascular
bed, septic shock

224 S Upper extremity procedures except humerus +
hand age < 70 without
DX 2

Potential for infection

225 S Foot procedures

Self-care deficit

226 S Soft tissue procedures
age > 69 and/or DX 2

Impaired physical mobility,
limb trauma

227 S Soft tissue procedures
age < 70 without DX 2

228 S Ganglion hand procedures

229 S Hand procedures except
ganglion

230 S Local excision + removal
of internal fixation devices
of hip + femur

231 S Local excision + removal
of internal fixation devices
except hip + femur

232 S Athroscopy

233 S Other musculoskeletal system + connective tissue O.R. procedures age > 69 and/or DX 2

234 S Other musculoskeletal system + connective tissue O.R. procedures age < 70 without DX 2

235 M Fractures of femur

236 M Fractures of hip + pelvis

237 M Sprains, strains + dislocations of hip, pelvis + thigh

238 M Osteomyelitis

239 M Pathological fractures + musculoskeletal system + connective tissue malignancy

240 M Connective tissue disorders age > 69 and/or DX 2

241 M Connective tissue disorders age < 70 without DX 2

242 M Septic arthritis

243 M Medical back problems

244 M Bone diseases + septic arthropathy age > 69 and/or DX 2

245 M Bone diseases + septic arthropathy age < 70 without DX 2

246 M Nonspecific arthropathies

247 M Signs + symptoms of musculoskeletal system + connective tissue

248 M Tendonitis, myositis + bursitis

249 M Aftercare, musculo-
skeletal system + connec-
tive tissue
250 M Fracture, sprains,
strains + dislocation of
forearm, hand, foot age
> 69 and/or DX 2
251 M Fracture, sprains,
strains + dislocation of
forearm, hand, foot age
18-69 without DX 2
252 M Fracture, sprains,
strains + dislocation of
forearm, hand, foot age
0-17
253 M Fracture, sprains,
strains + dislocation of
upper arm, lower leg,
except foot age > 69
and/or DX 2
254 M Fracture, sprains,
strains + dislocation of
upper arm, lower leg,
except foot age 18-69
without DX 2
255 M Fracture, sprains,
strains, + dislocation of
upper arm, lower leg,
except foot age 0-17
256 M Other diagnoses of
musculoskeletal system +
connective tissue

DISEASES OF THE SKIN, SUBCUTANEOUS TISSUE, AND BREAST

Major Diagnostic Categories DRG	Nursing Diagnostic Categories NDRG
257 S Total mastectomy for malignancy age > 69 and/or DX 2	Noncompliance Role disturbance

258 S Total mastectomy for age < 70 without DX 2 — Sexual dysfunction

259 S Subtotal mastectomy for malignancy age > 69 and/or DX 2 — Family process altered / Knowledge deficit / Health maintenance altered

260 S Subtotal mastectomy for malignancy age < 70 — Loneliness / Hopelessness

261 S Breast procedures for nonmalignancy except biopsy + local excision — Powerlessness / Anger

262 S Breast biopsy + local excision for nonmalignancy — Denial / Body image disturbance

263 S Skin grafts for skin ulcer or cellulitis age > 69 and/or DX 2 — Self-concept/self-esteem disturbance / Anxiety

264 S Skin grafts for skin ulcer or cellulitis age < 70 without DX 2 — Fear / Depression

265 S Skin grafts except for skin ulcer or cellulitis with DX 2 — Loss / Pain

266 S Skin grafts except for skin ulcer or cellulitis without DX 2 — Stress / Skin integrity impaired

267 S Perianal + pilonidal procedures — Actual plasma volume deficit, burn shock

268 S Skin, subcutaneous tissue + breast plastic procedures — Vasodilatation of vascular bed, septic shock

269 S Other skin, subcutaneous tissue + breast O.R. procedures age > 69 and/or DX 2 — Potential for infection / Self-care deficit

270 S Other skin, subcutaneous tissue + breast O.R. procedures age < 70 without DX 2

271 M Skin ulcers

272 M Major skin disorders age > 69 and/or DX 2

273 M Major skin disorders age < 70 without DX 2

274 M Malignant breast disorders age > 69 and/or DX 2

275 M Malignant breast disorders age < 70 without DX 2

276 M Nonmalignant breast disorders

277 M Cellulitis age > 69 and/or DX 2

278 M Cellulitis age 18-69 without DX 2

279 M Cellulitis age 0-17

280 M Trauma to the skin, subcutaneous tissue + breast age > 69 and/or DX 2

281 M Trauma to the skin, subcutaneous tissue + breast age 18-69 without DX 2

282 M Trauma to the skin, subcutaneous tissue + breast age 0-17

283 M Minor skin disorders age > 69 and/or DX 2

284 M Minor skin disorders age < 70 without DX 2

ENDOCRINE, NUTRITIONAL, AND METABOLIC DISEASES

Major Diagnostic Categories DRG	Nursing Diagnostic Categories NDRG
285 S Amputation for endocrine, nutritional + metabolic disorders	Thought process altered, confusion
286 S Adrenal + pituitary procedures	Noncompliance
	Role disturbance

287 S Skin grafts + wound debridement for endocrine, nutritional + metabolic disorders

Violence directed toward others

Violence directed toward self

288 S O.R. procedures for obesity

Sexual dysfunction

289 S Parathyroid procedures

Knowledge deficit

290 S Thyroid procedures

Activity intolerance

291 S Thyroglossal procedures

Psychological immobility

292 S Other endocrine, nutritional + metabolic O.R. procedures age > 70 and/or DX 2

Impaired physical mobility, muscular weakness

293 S Other endocrine, nutritional + metabolic O.R. age < 70 without DX 2

Hopelessness

Depersonalization

294 M Diabetes age ≥ 36

Powerlessness

295 M Diabetes age 0–35

Anger

296 M Nutritional + miscellaneous metabolic disorders age > 69 and/or DX 2

Denial

Body image disturbance

297 M Nutritional + miscellaneous metabolic disorders age 18–69 without DX 2

Anxiety

Fear

298 M Nutritional + miscellaneous metabolic disorders age 0–17

Loss

Depression

299 M Inborn errors of metabolism

Pain

300 M Endocrine disorders age > 69 and/or DX 2

Sensory deprivation

301 M Endocrine disorders age < 70 without DX 2

Sleep deprivation

Skin integrity impaired

Potential for infection

Self-care deficit

Extracellular fluid volume excess, edema

Intracellular electrolyte excess, hyperkalemia

Intracellular electrolyte deficit, hypokalemia

Extracellular electrolyte
excess, hypernatremia
Extracellular electrolyte
deficit, hyponatremia
Intracellular electrolyte
excess, hypermagnesium
Intracellular electrolyte
deficit, hypomagnesium
Acid–base imbalance, metabolic acidosis
Acid–base imbalance, metabolic alkalosis
Bowel elimination decreased,
constipation
Bowel elimination increased,
diarrhea
Nutritional alteration, less
than body requirements
Nutritional alteration, more
than body requirements
Arrhythmias (see "Circulatory
System" section in this
chapter)

DISEASES AND DISORDERS OF THE KIDNEYS AND URINARY TRACT

Major Diagnostic Categories DRG	Nursing Diagnosis Categories NDRG
302 S Kidney transplant	Extracellular fluid volume excess, edema
303 S Kidney, ureter + major bladder procedures for neoplasms	Intracellular electrolyte excess, hyperkalemia
304 S Kidney, ureter + major bladder procedures for nonmalignant age > 69 and/or DX 2	Intracellular electrolyte deficit, hypokalemia

305 S Kidney, ureter + major bladder procedures for nonmalignant age < 70 without DX 2 — Extracellular electrolyte excess, hypernatremia

306 S Prostatectomy age > 69 and/or DX 2 — Extracellular electrolyte deficit, hyponatremia

307 S Prostatectomy age < 70 without DX 2

308 S Minor bladder procedures age > 69 and/or DX 2 — Intracellular electrolyte excess hypermagnesium

309 S Minor bladder procedures age < 70 without DX 2 — Intracellular electrolyte deficit, hypomagnesium

310 S Transurethral procedures age > 69 and/or DX 2 — Actual whole blood volume deficit, hemorrhagic shock

311 S Transurethral procedures age < 70 without DX 2 — Renal tissue perfusion decreased

Actual whole blood and plasma volume deficit, traumatic shock

312 S Urethral procedures, age > 69 and/or DX 2 — Urinary output decreased, oliguria

313 S Urethral procedures, age 18–69 without DX 2 — Urinary output increased, polyuria

314 S Urethral procedures, age 0–17 — Actual fluid volume and electrolyte deficit, diabetic shock

315 S Other kidney + urinary tract O.R. procedures — Acid–base imbalance, metabolic acidosis

316 M Renal failure without dialysis — Acid–base imbalance, metabolic alkalosis

317 M Renal failure with dialysis — Thought process altered, confusion

318 M Kidney + urinary tract neoplasms age > 69 and/or DX 2 — Violence directed toward others

Noncompliance

319 M Kidney + urinary tract neoplasms age < 70 without DX 2 — Diversional activity deficit

Role disturbance

320 M Kidney + urinary tract infections age > 69 and/or DX 2

Family process altered
Knowledge deficit

321 M Kidney + urinary tract infections age 18–69 without DX 2

Impaired physical mobility, muscular weakness

322 M Kidney + urinary tract infections age 0–17

Activity intolerance
Hopelessness

323 M Urinary stones age > 69 and/or DX 2

Powerlessness

324 M Urinary stones age < 70 without DX 2

Anger

325 M Kidney + urinary tract signs + symptoms age > 69 and/or DX 2

Denial
Body image disturbance

326 M Kidney + urinary tract signs + symptoms age 18–69 without DX 2

Anxiety
Fear

327 M Kidney + urinary tract signs + symptoms age 0–17

Depression
Loss

328 M Urethral strictures age > 69 and/or DX 2

Pain

329 M Urethral stricture age 18–69 without DX 2

Sensory overload

330 M Urethral stricture age 0–17

Sensory deprivation

331 M Other kidney + urinary tract diagnoses age > 69 and/or DX 2

Stress
Sleep deprivation

332 M Other kidney + urinary tract diagnoses age 18–69 without DX 2

Alteration in right ventricular-atrial preload

333 M Other kidney + urinary tract diagnoses age 0–17

Alteration in left ventricular-atrial preload
Cardiac output decreased
Arterial blood pressure altered, hypotension
Arterial blood pressure altered, hypertension

Arrhythmias (see "Circulatory
  System" section in this
  chapter)
Extracellular fluid volume
  excess, alveolar edema
Oxygen–carbon dioxide gas
  exchange imbalance,
  crackles
Bowel elimination decreased,
  constipation
Bowel elimination increased,
  diarrhea
Nutritional alteration, less
  than body requirements
Nutritional alteration, more
  than body requirements
Oral mucous membrane,
  alteration in
Skin integrity impaired
Self-care deficit

DISEASES AND DISORDERS OF THE MALE REPRODUCTIVE SYSTEM

Major Diagnostic Categories DRG	Nursing Diagnostic Categories NDRG
334 S Major male pelvic procedures with DX 2	Role disturbance
335 S Major male pelvic procedures without DX 2	Sexual dysfunction
336 S Transurethral prostatectomy age > 69 and/or DX 2	Knowledge deficit Anger
337 S Transurethral prostatectomy age 70 without DX 2	Denial Body image disturbance
338 Testes procedures for malignancy	Anxiety

339 S Testes procedures, nonmalignant age > 17
340 S Testes procedures, nonmalignant age 0–17
341 S Penis procedures

342 S Circumcision age > 17
343 S Circumcision age 0–17
344 S Other male repro-
   ductive system O.R. procedures for malignancy
345 S Other male reproductive system O.R. procedures
   except for malignancy
346 M Malignancy, male
   reproductive system, age
   > 69 and/or DX 2
347 M Malignancy, male
   reproductive system, age
   < 70 without DX 2
348 M Benign prostatic
   hypertrophy age > 69
   and/or DX 2
349 M Benign prostatic
   hypertrophy age < 70
   without DX 2
350 M Inflammation of the
   male reproduction system
351 M Sterilization, male
352 M Other male reproductive system diagnoses

Fear
Pain
Stress
Potential for infection
Urinary output decreased,
   oliguria
Self-care deficit

DISEASES AND DISORDERS OF THE FEMALE REPRODUCTIVE SYSTEM

Major Diagnostic Categories
DRG

353 S Pelvic evisceration,
   radical hysterectomy +
   vulvectomy

Nursing Diagnostic Categories
NDRG

Noncompliance
Role disturbance

354 S Nonradical hyster-
  ectomy age > 69 and/or
  DX 2

Sexual dysfunction
Knowledge deficit

355 S Nonradical hyster-
  ectomy age < 70 without
  DX 2

Hopelessness
Powerlessness

356 S Female reproductive
  system reconstructive
  procedures

Anger
Denial

357 S Uterus + adenexa procedures, for malignancy

Self-concept/self-esteem disturbance
Body-image disturbance

358 S Uterus + adenexa procedures for nonmalignancy
  except tubal interruption

Anxiety
Fear

359 S Tubal interruption for
  nonmalignancy

Loss

360 S Vagina, cervix + vulva
  procedures

Pain

361 S Laparoscopy + endo-
  scopy (female) except
  tubal interruption

Stress
Skin integrity impaired

362 S Laparoscopic tubal
  interruption

Potential for infection

363 S D & C, conization +
  radiological implant, for
  malignancy

364 S D & C, conization
  except for malignancy

365 S Other female repro-
  ductive system O.R. procedures

366 M Malignancy, female
  reproductive system age
  > 69 and/or DX 2

367 M Malignancy, female
  reproductive system age
  < 70 without DX 2

368 M Infections, female
  reproductive system

369 M Menstrual + other
  female reproductive system disorders

PREGNANCY, CHILDBIRTH, AND THE PUERPERIUM

Major Diagnostic Categories DRG	Nursing Diagnostic Categories NDRG
370 S Cesarean section with DX 2	Noncompliance
371 S Cesarean section without DX 2	Role disturbance
372 M Vaginal delivery with complicating diagnosis	Sexual dysfunction
	Family process altered
373 M Vaginal delivery without complicating diagnoses	Knowledge deficit
	Activity intolerance
374 S Vaginal delivery with sterilization and/or D & C	Loneliness
	Hopelessness
375 S Vaginal delivery with O.R. procedures except sterilization and/or D & C	Anger
	Denial
376 M Postpartum diagnoses without O.R. procedures	Body-image disturbance
377 S Postpartum diagnoses with O.R. procedures	Anxiety
378 M Ectopic pregnancy	Fear
379 M Threatened abortion	Depression
380 M Abortion without D & C	Loss
381 M Abortion with D & C	Pain
382 M False labor	Stress
383 M Other antepartum diagnoses with medical complications	Potential for infection
	Skin integrity impaired
384 M Other antepartum diagnoses without medical complications	Self-care deficit

NORMAL NEWBORNS AND OTHER NEONATES WITH CERTAIN CONDITIONS ORIGINATING IN THE PERINATAL PERIOD

Major Diagnostic Categories DRG	Nursing Diagnostic Categories NDRG
385 S Neonates, died or transferred	To be developed
386 S Extreme immaturity, neonate	
387 S Combined with 388	
388 S Prematurity with and without major problems	
389 S Full-term neonate with major problems	
390 S Neonates with other significant problems	
391 S Normal newborns	

DISEASES OF THE SKIN, SUBCUTANEOUS TISSUE, AND BREAST

Major Diagnostic Categories DRG	Nursing Diagnostic Categories NDRG
392 S Splenectomy age > 17	Noncompliance
393 S Splenectomy age 0–17	Knowledge deficit
394 S Other O.R. procedures of the blood + blood-forming organs	Activity intolerance Hopelessness
395 M Red blood cell disorders age > 17	Powerlessness
396 M Red blood cell disorders age 0–17	Anger
397 M Coagulation disorders	Denial
398 M Reticuloendothelial + immunity disorders age > 69 and/or DX 2	Fear Depression

399 M Reticuloendothelial +
immunity disorders age
< 70 without DX 2

Pain
Peripheral tissue perfusion
obstructed, thrombo-
phlebitis
Actual whole blood volume
deficit, hemorrhagic shock
Potential for infection
Skin integrity impaired
Self-care deficit

MYELOPROLIFERATIVE DISORDERS AND POORLY-DIFFERENTIATED MALIGNANCIES AND OTHER NEOPLASMS

**Major Diagnostic Categories
DRG**

**Nursing Diagnostic Categories
NDRG**

400 S Lymphoma or leukemia
with major O.R. proce-
dures
401 S Lymphoma or leukemia
with minor O.R. proce-
dures age > 69 and/or
DX 2
402 S Lymphoma or leukemia
with minor O.R. proce-
dures age < 70 without
DX 2
403 M Lymphoma or leukemia
age > 69 and/or DX 2
404 M Lymphoma or leukemia
age 18–69 without DX 2
405 M Lymphoma or leukemia
age 0–17
406 S Myeloproliferative disorders or poorly differ-
entiated neoplasms with
major O.R. procedures
and/or DX 2

Thought process altered, con-
fusion
Noncompliance
Diversional activity deficit
Role disturbance

Sexual dysfunction
Impaired physical mobility,
muscular weakness

Psychological immobility
Activity intolerance
Hopelessness

Depersonalization
Powerlessness

407 S Myeloproliferative disorders or poorly differentiated neoplasms with major O.R. procedures without DX 2

Anger
Denial

408 S Myeloproliferative disorders or poorly differentiated neoplasms with minor O.R. procedures

Body-image disturbance
Anxiety

409 M Radiotherapy

Fear

410 M Chemotherapy

Depression

411 M History of malignancy without endoscopy

Loss

412 M History of malignancy with endoscopy

Pain

413 M Other myeloproliferative disorders or poorly differentiated neoplasms DX age > 69 and/or DX 2

Stress
Sensory deprivation

414 M Other myeloproliferative disorders or poorly differentiated neoplasms DX age < 70 without DX 2

Sleep deprivation
Arterial blood pressure, hypotension
Extracellular fluid volume excess, alveolar edema
Ineffective breathing pattern, dyspnea
Oxygen–carbon dioxide gas exchange impaired, crackles
Extracellular fluid volume excess, edema
Nutritional alteration, less than body requirements
Skin integrity impaired
Self-care deficit

INFECTIOUS AND PARASITIC DISEASES (SYSTEMIC)

Major Diagnostic Categories DRG	Nursing Diagnostic Categories NDRG
415 S O.R. procedure for infectious + parasitic diseases	Potential for infection Knowledge deficit

416 M Septicemia age > 17
417 M Septicemia age 0–17
418 M Postoperative + post-
traumatic infections

419 M Fever of unknown
origin > 69 and/or DX 2
420 M Fever of unknown
origin age 18–69 without
DX 2

421 M Viral illness age > 17
422 M Viral illness + fever of
unknown origin age 0–17
423 M Other infectious +
parasitic disease diagnoses

Anxiety
Fear
Pain
Acid–base imbalance, meta-
bolic acidosis
Nutritional alteration, less
than body requirements
Nutritional alteration, more
than body requirements
Vasodilatation of vascular
bed, septic shock
Skin integrity impaired
Arterial blood pressure
altered, hypotension
Self-care deficit

MENTAL DISORDERS

Major Diagnostic Categories DRG	Nursing Diagnostic Categories NDRG
424 S O.R. procedures with principal diagnosis of mental illness	Verbal/nonverbal communi- cation deficit Verbal/nonverbal communi- cation excess
425 M Acute adjustment re- actions + disturbances of psychosocial dysfunction	Violence directed toward self Violence directed toward others Noncompliance
426 M Depressive neuroses	Knowledge deficit
427 M Neuroses except de- pressive	Loneliness
428 M Disorders of person- ality + impulse control	Hopelessness Anxiety
429 M Organic disturbances + mental retardation	Fear Depression
430 M Psychoses	Depersonalization
431 M Childhood mental dis- orders	Psychological immobility
432 M Other diagnoses of mental disorders	Denial Self-care deficit Self-concept/self-esteem dis- turbance

SUBSTANCE USE DISORDERS AND SUBSTANCE-INDUCED ORGANIC DISORDERS

Major Diagnostic Categories DRG	Nursing Diagnostic Categories NDRG
433 S Combined with 434–438 (discharged against medical advice not in MEDPAR set)	Thought process altered, confusion
	Verbal/nonverbal communication deficit
434 S Drug dependence	Verbal/nonverbal communication excess
435 S Drug use except dependence	Noncompliance
436 S Alcohol dependence	Knowledge deficit
437 S Alcohol use except dependence	Family process altered
438 S Alcohol + substance-induced organic mental syndrome	Violence directed toward others
	Violence directed toward self
	Hopelessness
	Loneliness
	Denial
	Anger
	Anxiety
	Fear
	Depression
	Stress
	Thought process altered, loss of consciousness
	Self-care deficit
	Body-image disturbance
	Self-concept/self-esteem disturbance

INJURY, POISONING, AND TOXIC EFFECTS OF DRUGS

Major Diagnostic Categories DRG	Nursing Diagnostic Categories NDRG
439 S Skin grafts for injuries	Knowledge deficit
440 S Wound debridements for injuries	Powerlessness
441 S Head procedures for injuries	Hopelessness
442 S Other O.R. procedures for injuries age > 69 and/or DX 2	Anger Denial
443 S Other O.R. procedures for injuries age < 70 without DX 2	Anxiety Fear
444 M Multiple trauma age > 69 and/or DX 2	Loss Pain
445 M Multiple trauma age 18–69	Body-image disturbance
446 M Multiple trauma age 0–17	Stress
447 M Allergic reactions age > 17	Sensory deprivation
449 M Allergic reactions age 0–17	See "Circulatory System" NDRG, pp. 410–414
449 M Toxic effects of drugs age > 69 and/or DX 2	See "Kidney and Urinary Tract" NDRG, pp. 427–430
	See "Nervous System" NDRG, pp. 403–405
450 M Toxic effects of drugs age 18–69 without DX 2	See "Respiratory System" NDRG, pp. 408–410
451 M Toxic effects of drugs age 0–17	Skin integrity impaired deficit, burn shock
452 M Complications of treatment age > 69 and/or DX 2	Potential for infection

453 M Complications of treatment age < 70 without DX 2
454 M Other injuries, poisonings + toxic effects of drugs age > 69 and/or DX 2
455 M Other injuries, poisonings + toxic effects of drugs age < 70 without DX 2

BURNS

Major Diagnostic Categories DRG	Nursing Diagnostic Categories NDRG
456 S Combined with 457–460 (discharged against medical advice not in MEDPAR set)	See "Circulatory System" NDRG, pp. 410–414
457 S Extensive burns	See "Kidney and Urinary Tract" NDRG, pp. 427–430
458 S Nonextensive burns with skin grafts	See "Respiratory System" NDRG, pp. 408–410
	Role disturbance
459 S Nonextensive burns with wound debridement + O.R. procedures	Family process altered
	Sexual dysfunction
460 M Nonextensive burns without O.R. procedures	Activity intolerance
	Psychological immobility
	Loneliness
	Hopelessness
	Powerlessness
	Anger
	Denial
	Anxiety
	Fear
	Body-image disturbance
	Self-concept/self-esteem disturbance
	Loss

Depression
Pain
Sensory deprivations
Sensory overload
Skin integrity impaired
Potential for infection
Knowledge deficit
Self-care deficit

SELECTED FACTORS INFLUENCING HEALTH STATUS AND CONTACT WITH HEALTH SERVICES

Major Diagnostic Categories DRG	Nursing Diagnostic Categories NDRG
461 S O.R. procedures with diagnoses of other contact with health services	Knowledge deficit Noncompliance
462 M Rehabilitation	Impaired physical mobility, hemiparesis
463 M Signs + symptoms with DX 2	Impaired physical mobility, hemiplegia
464 M Signs + symptoms without DX 2	Depression
465 M Combined with 466	Pain
466 M Aftercare with and without history of malignancy as DX 2	Anxiety Denial
467 M Other factors influencing health status	Self-care deficit

REFERENCES

Dowling, W. Prospective rate setting: Concept and practice. *Top Health Care Finances*, 3, 7–37, 1976.

Erickson, S. DRGs: expanding nursing responsibilities in the CCU. *Dimensions in Critical Care Nursing*, 4(2), 103–109.

Grimaldi, P. & Micheletti, J. *Diagnosis Related Groups: A Practitioner's Guide*. Chicago: Pluribus Press, 1983.

Kelly, M. *Nursing diagnosis sourcebook*. Norwalk, Conn.: Appleton-Century-Crofts, 1985.

Levine, E. & Abdellah F. DRGs: A recent refinement to an old method. *Inquiry*, 21, 105–112, Summer 1984.

Lindammod, M. DRGs: Potential effects on critical care nursing. *Dimension of Critical Care Nursing*, (4)2, 92–99, March–April 1985.

Shaffer, F. A. DRGs: History and review. *Topics of Health Record Management*, 15–34, 1984.

Smith, C. DRG: Making them work for you. *Nursing '85*, (15)1, 34–41, January 1985.

Wake, M., McLane, A., & Gatch, P. Nursing diagnosis in critical care: Reflections and future direction. *Heart & Lung*, 14(5), 444–448, September 1985.

8

Defining Characteristics and Possible Nursing Diagnostic Categories or Groups

REGULATORY BEHAVIORS

ABDOMINAL CRAMPS/PAIN

R/O*
  Loss
  Vasodilatation of vascular bed, anaphylactic shock
  Intra-abdominal perfusion, decreased
  Nutritional alteration, less than body requirements
  Glucose excess, hyperglycemia
  Bowel elimination, decreased, constipation
  Bowel elimination, increased, diarrhea
  Bowel elimination, uncontrolled, incontinence

ACTIVITY TOLERANCE, DECREASED

R/O
  Cardiac output, decreased
  Peripheral tissue perfusion, decreased

*R/O = rule out

Extracellular fluid volume excess, alveolar edema
Nutritional alteration, less than body requirements

ANOREXIA

R/O

Psychological immobility
Self-concept–self-esteem disturbance
Body-image disturbance
Fear
Depression
Sensory overload
Alteration right ventricular–atrial preload
Actual fluid volume electrolyte deficit, diabetic shock
Serum glucose excess, hyperglycemia

ARRHYTHMIAS

R/O

Thought process, altered, confusion
Activity intolerance
Denial
Anxiety
Cardiac output, increased
Vasodilatation of vascular bed, anaphylactic shock
Oxygen–gas exchange, impaired, hypoxemia
Acid–base imbalance, respiratory acidosis
Vasodilatation of vascular bed, neurogenic shock
Intracellular electrolyte deficit, hypokalemia
Acid–base imbalance, metabolic alkalosis

ASCITES

R/O

Alteration in right ventricular–atrial preload

ASTERIXIS

R/O

Carbon dioxide gas exchange, impaired, hypercapnia

ATAXIA

R/O
  Intracranial pressure, increased

AUDITORY COMPREHENSION, DECREASED

R/O
  Verbal/nonverbal communication deficit
  Depersonalization
  Thought process, altered, level of consciousness reduced

AURA

R/O
  Central nervous system (CNS) altered, seizure

BABINSKI'S SIGN

R/O
  Impaired physical mobility, hemiparesis
  Intracranial pressure, increased

BRADYCARDIA

R/O
  Intracranial pressure, increased
  Extracellular volume excess, cerebral edema

BREATHLESSNESS

R/O
  Ineffective breathing pattern, dyspnea

BOWEL SOUNDS DECREASED

R/O
  Bowel elimination, decreased, constipation

CATECHOLAMINES, INCREASED

R/O
  Stress

Sensory deprivation
REM sleep deprivation

CARDIAC OUTPUT, DECREASED

R/O
   Atrial conduction, altered, paroxysmal atrial tachycardia
      (PAT)
   Atrial conduction, altered, atrial flutter
   Atrial conduction, altered, atrial fibrillation
   Atrial-ventricular conduction, altered, premature junctional
      beat
   Ventricular conduction, altered, premature ventricular beat
   Ventricular conduction, altered, accelerated idioventricular
      rhythm
   Alteration in cardiopulmonary stability, chest injury shock
   Vasodilatation of vascular bed, anaphylactic shock
   Ineffective breathing pattern, alveolar hypoventilation
   Vasodilatation of vascular bed, neurogenic shock
   Actual plasma volume deficit, burn shock

CARDIAC OUTPUT, INCREASED

R/O
   Stress

CEREBRAL BLOOD FLOW, INCREASED

R/O
   Sensory overload

CEREBRAL BLOOD FLOW, REDUCED

R/O
   Extracellular volume excess, cerebral edema

CEREBROVASCULAR RESISTANCE, INCREASED

R/O
   Extracellular volume excess, cerebral edema

CHANGE IN RESPIRATORY PATTERN

R/O
   Intracranial pressure, increased
   Extracellular fluid volume excess, cerebral edema
   Actual fluid volume and electrolyte deficit, diabetic shock
   Serum glucose excess, hyperglycemia

CHEST PAIN/ANGINA

R/O
   Sexual dysfunction
   Activity intolerance
   Denial
   Anxiety
   Cardiac output, decreased
   Cerebral artery perfusion, decreased
   Sinus conduction, altered, sinus tachycardia
   Atrial conduction, altered, PAT
   Atrial conduction, altered, atrial flutter
   Atrial conduction, altered, atrial fibrillation
   Atrial–ventricular conduction, altered, junctional tachy-
      cardia
   Atrial–ventricular conduction, altered, complete heart
      block
   Ventricular conduction, altered, premature ventricular beat
   Ventricular conduction, altered, ventricular tachycardia
   Ventricular conduction, altered, ventricular fibrillation
   Alteration in distributive gas exchange, spontaneous
      pneumothorax
   Swallowing pattern, altered, dysphagia

CHEYNE-STOKES

R/O
   Alteration in left ventricular–atrial preload

CLONUS

R/O
   CNS altered, seizure

COMA

R/O

Thought process, altered, level of consciousness altered
Cerebral tissue perfusion, decreased
Cerebral perfusion, obstructed, thromboembolism
Intracellular electrolyte deficit, hypokalemia
Extracellular electrolyte deficit, hyponatremia
Acid–base imbalance, metabolic alkalosis

CONSTIPATION

R/O

Depression

CONVULSION

R/O

Arterial blood pressure, altered, hypertension
Ventricular conduction, altered, ventricular fibrillation
Extracellular electrolyte excess, hypernatremia
Extracellular electrolyte deficit, hyponatremia
Actual whole blood and plasma volume deficit, traumatic
    shock
Serum glucose deficit, hypoglycemia

COOL EXTREMITIES

R/O

Alteration in right ventricular–atrial preload
Cardiac output, decreased
Arterial blood pressure, altered, hypotension
Peripheral tissue perfusion, decreased
Systemic vascular resistance, altered, afterload
Sinus conduction, altered, sinus tachycardia
Atrial conduction, altered, atrial fibrillation
Intracellular fluid volume deficit, dehydration
Actual whole blood volume deficit, hemorrhagic shock
Vasodilatation of vascular bed, septic shock

CORONARY VASOCONSTRICTION

R/O

Stress

COUGH

R/O

Extracellular fluid volume excess, alveolar edema
Oxygen–carbon dioxide gas exchange, impaired, crackles
Alteration in distributive gas exchange, spontaneous pneumothorax

CENTRAL VENOUS PRESSURE, DECREASED

R/O

Intracellular fluid volume deficit, dehydration

CENTRAL VENOUS PRESSURE, INCREASED

R/O

Systemic vascular resistance, altered, afterload
Cardiac output, decreased
Cardiac output, increased
Actual reduction in cardiac output, cardiogenic shock
Extracellular fluid volume excess, edema
Renal tissue perfusion, decreased
Vasodilatation of vascular bed, septic shock

CYANOSIS

R/O

Activity intolerance
Alteration in right ventricular–atrial preload
Systemic vascular resistance, altered, afterload
Peripheral tissue perfusion, decreased
Obstructed peripheral tissue perfusion, thromboembolism
Atrial conduction, altered, atrial fibrillation
Ventricular conduction, altered, ventricular fibrillation
Alteration in cardiopulmonary stability, chest injury shock
Actual reduction in cardiac output, cardiogenic shock
Vasodilatation of vascular bed, anaphylactic shock
Extracellular fluid volume excess, alveolar edema
Oxygen–gas exchange, impaired, hypoxemia
Carbon dioxide gas exchange, impaired, hypercapnia
Acid–base imbalance, respiratory acidosis
Pulmonary tissue perfusion, altered, emboli

Alteration in distributive gas exchange, spontaneous pneumothorax
Ventilation–perfusion imbalance
Actual whole blood and plasma volume deficit, traumatic
  shock

DEAFNESS

R/O
Verbal/nonverbal communication deficit

DIAPHORESIS

R/O
Thought process, altered, confusion
Verbal/nonverbal communication excess
Activity intolerance
Anger
Anxiety
Fear
Pain
Cardiac output, increased
Coronary artery perfusion, decreased
Extracellular fluid volume excess, alveolar edema
Acid–base imbalance, respiratory acidosis
Intracellular fluid volume deficit, dehydration

DIARRHEA

R/O
Depression
Cardiac output, increased
Vasodilatation of vascular bed, anaphylactic shock
Intracellular electrolyte excess, hyperkalemia
Intra-abdominal perfusion, decreased

DIFFICULTY PERFORMING ROLE

R/O
Role disturbance

DILATION OF BRONCHIOLES

R/O
   Anxiety
   Stress

DIZZINESS

R/O
   Activity intolerance
   Depersonalization
   Powerlessness
   Fear
   Cardiac output, decreased
   Sinus conduction, altered, sinus arrhythmia
   Sinus conduction, altered, sinus bradycardia
   Sinus conduction, altered, sinus pause or block
   Sinus conduction, altered, sinus atrial exit block
   Atrial–ventricular conduction, alterated, Mobitz Type I
   Atrial–ventricular conduction, alterated, Mobitz Type II
   Ventricular conduction, altered, ventricular tachycardia
   Ventricular conduction, altered, idioventricular accelerated
      rhythm
   Cardiopulmonary stability, altered, chest injury shock
   Cerebral tissue perfusion, decreased
   Cerebral tissue perfusion, obstructed, thromboembolism
   Vasodilatation of vascular bed, neurogenic shock
   Actual whole blood volume deficit, hemorrhagic shock
   Actual fluid volume and electrolyte deficit, diabetic shock

DRY MOUTH

R/O
   Anxiety
   Fear
   Depression
   Intracellular fluid volume deficit, dehydration

DYSPNEA

R/O
   Sexual dysfunction

Activity intolerance
Stress
Alteration in atrial–ventricular preload
Systemic vascular resistance, altered, afterload
Cardiac output, decreased
Cardiac output, increased
Sinus conduction, altered, sinus tachycardia
Atrial conduction, altered, atrial flutter
Atrial conduction, altered, atrial fibrillation
Atrial–ventricular conduction, altered, Mobitz Type I
Atrial–ventricular conduction, altered, Mobitz Type II
Atrial-ventricular conduction, altered, complete heart block
Ventricular conduction, altered, accelerated idioventricular
    rhythm
Alteration in cardiopulmonary stability, chest injury shock
Actual reduction in cardiac output, cardiogenic shock
Vasodilatation of vascular bed, anaphylactic shock
Extracellular fluid volume excess, alveolar edema
Acid–base imbalance, respiratory acidosis
Ineffective breathing pattern, alveolar hyperventilation
Oxygen–carbon dioxide gas exchange, impaired, crackles
Ineffective airway clearance, wheezes
Pulmonary tissue perfusion, altered, emboli
Altered distributive gas exchange, spontaneous pneumo-
    thorax
Ventilation–perfusion imbalance
Renal tissue perfusion, decreased

EDEMA

R/O

Altered right ventricular–atrial preload
Peripheral tissue perfusion, decreased
Actual reduction in cardiac output, cardiogenic shock
Vasodilatation of vascular bed, anaphylactic shock
Pulmonary tissue perfusion, altered, emboli
Vasodilatation of vascular bed, neurogenic shock
Renal tissue perfusion, decreased
Urinary output, decreased, oliguria
Extracellular fluid volume excess, intrapleural edema or
    ascites

FACIAL WEAKNESS

R/O
Impaired physical mobility, hemiparesis

FAINTING

R/O
Pain
Sinus conduction, altered, sinus bradycardia
Sinus conduction, altered, sinus pause or block
Sinus conduction, altered, sinoatrial (SA) exit block
Atrial–ventricular conduction, altered, Mobitz Type II
Atrial–ventricular conduction, altered, complete heart block

FATIGUE

R/O
Psychological immobility
Loneliness
Depersonalization
Powerlessness
Fear
Depression
Systemic vascular resistance, altered, afterload
Cardiac output, decreased
Atrial conduction, altered, premature atrial contractions (PAC)
Atrial conduction, altered, atrial flutter
Atrial conduction, altered, atrial fibrillation
Atrial–ventricular conduction, altered, junctional tachycardia
Atrial–ventricular conduction, altered, Mobitz Type I
Atrial–ventricular conduction, altered, Mobitz Type II
Ineffective breathing pattern, alveolar hyperventilation
Ineffective breathing pattern, dyspnea
Oxygen–carbon dioxide gas exchange, impaired, crackles
Ineffective airway clearance, wheezes
Ventilation–perfusion imbalance
Intracellular fluid volume deficit, dehydration
Intracellular electrolyte excess, hyperkalemia
Renal tissue perfusion, decreased

FEVER

R/O
   Impaired physical mobility, hemiplegia
   Bowel elimination, increased, diarrhea
   Intra-abdominal perfusion, decreased

NERVOUSNESS

R/O
   Sensory overload

FLUSHING

R/O
   Anxiety
   Serum glucose excess, hyperglycemia

HEADACHE

R/O
   Impaired physical mobility, hemiplegia
   Powerlessness
   Depression
   Altered arterial blood pressure, hypertension
   Oxygen gas exchange, impaired, hypoxemia
   Carbon dioxide exchange, impaired, hypercapnia
   Intracranial pressure, increased
   CNS altered, seizure
   Extracellular fluid volume excess, cerebral edema
   Cerebral tissue perfusion, decreased
   Cerebral tissue perfusion, obstructed
   Extracellular electrolyte deficit, hyponatremia
   Bowel elimination, decreased, constipation
   Serum glucose deficit, hypoglycemia

HEPATOMEGALY

R/O
   Alteration in right ventricular–atrial preload
   Serum glucose excess, hyperglycemia

HYPERACTIVE TENDON REFLEXES

R/O
  Impaired physical mobility, hemiparesis
  Acid–base imbalance, metabolic alkalosis

HYPERTENSION

R/O
  Thought process, altered, confusion
  Verbal/nonverbal communication excess
  Impaired physical mobility, hemiplegia
  Anger
  Denial
  Self-concept/self-esteem disturbance
  Body-image disturbance
  Anxiety
  Loss
  Stress
  REM sleep deprivation
  Oxygen gas exchange, impaired, hypoxemia
  Extracellular fluid volume excess, cerebral edema
  Extracellular fluid volume excess, edema

HYPERVENTILATION

R/O
  Sensory overload

HYPOTENSION

R/O
  Impaired physical mobility, hemiplegia
  Pain
  Cardiac output, decreased
  Coronary artery perfusion, decreased
  Atrial–ventricular conduction, altered, Mobitz Type II
  Ventricular conduction, altered, ventricular tachycardia
  Ventricular conduction, altered, accelerated idioventricular
    rhythm
  Alteration in cardiopulmonary stability, chest injury shock
  Actual reduction in cardiac output, cardiogenic shock

Vasodilatation of vascular bed, anaphylactic shock
Extracellular fluid volume excess, alveolar edema
Oxygen gas exchange, impaired, hypoxemia
Carbon dioxide gas exchange, impaired, hypercapnia
Ineffective breathing pattern, alveolar hypoventilation
Alteration in distributive gas exchange, spontaneous pneumothorax
Ventilation–perfusion imbalance
Vasodilatation of vascular bed, neurogenic shock
Intracellular fluid volume deficit, dehydration
Intracellular electrolyte deficit, hypokalemia
Actual whole blood and plasma volume deficit, traumatic shock
Intra-abdominal perfusion, decreased
Actual plasma volume deficit, burn shock

HYPOVENTILATION

R/O
Sensory overload

IMPAIRED MOBILITY

R/O
Injury, limb trauma
Injury, spinal trauma

INCONTINENCE

R/O
Thought process, altered, confusion
Ventricular conduction, altered, ventricular fibrillation
Cerebral perfusion, obstructed, thromboembolism

INDIGESTION

R/O
Depression

INSOMNIA

R/O
Diversional activity deficit

Fear
Depression

ITCHING/PURITUS

R/O
Vasodilatation of vascular bed, anaphylactic shock
Skin integrity, impaired

JOINT PAIN

R/O
Sexual dysfunction

MOTOR ACTIVITY, INCREASED

R/O
Violence directed toward others
Violence directed toward self

MUSCLE STRENGTH, DECREASED

R/O
Noncompliance

MUSCLE TENSION

R/O
Verbal/nonverbal communication deficit
Anger
Fear
Pain
Stress
Sensory overload

MYOCARDIAL CONTRACTION, INCREASED

R/O
Stress

NAUSEA

R/O
Anger

Anxiety
Fear
Depression
Pain
Alteration in left ventricular–atrial preload
Alteration in blood pressure, hypertension
Intracellular electrolyte deficit, hypokalemia
Actual fluid-volume and electrolyte deficit, diabetic shock
Bowel elimination, decreased, constipation
Serum glucose excess, hyperglycemia
Serum glucose deficit, hypoglycemia

NUMBNESS OF BODY PART

R/O
Psychological immobility
Depersonalization
Self-concept/self-esteem disturbance
Body-image disturbance
Sensory overload
Sensory deprivation
Arterial blood pressure, altered, hypertension
Acid–base imbalance, respiratory alkalosis
Cerebral perfusion, obstructed, thromboembolism

OLIGURIA

R/O
Stress
NREM sleep deprivation
Alteration in left ventricular–atrial preload
Systemic vascular resistance, altered, afterload
Cardiac output, decreased
Arterial blood pressure, altered, hypotension
Coronary artery perfusion, decreased
Sinus conduction, altered, sinus tachycardia
Actual reduction in cardiac output, cardiogenic shock
Vasodilatation of vascular bed, neurogenic shock
Intracellular fluid volume deficit, dehydration
Actual whole blood volume deficit, hemorrhagic shock
Renal tissue perfusion, decreased

Actual whole blood and plasma volume deficit, traumatic shock

Actual plasma volume deficit, burn shock

PALLOR

R/O

Activity intolerance

Pain

Systemic vascular resistance, altered, afterload

Arterial blood pressure, altered, hypotension

Arterial blood pressure, altered, hypertension

Peripheral tissue perfusion, decreased

Actual reduction in cardiac output, cardiogenic shock

Actual whole blood volume deficit, hemorrhagic shock

Renal tissue perfusion, decreased

Actual whole blood and plasma volume deficit, traumatic shock

Serum glucose deficit, hypoglycemia

PALPITATIONS

R/O

Sinus conduction, altered, sinus arrhythmias

Sinus conduction, altered, sinus bradycardia

Sinus conduction, altered, sinus pause or block

Sinus conduction, altered, SA exit block

Atrial conduction, altered, PAC

Atrial conduction, altered, PAT

Atrial conduction, altered, atrial flutter

Atrial conduction, altered, atrial fibrillation

Atrial-ventricular conduction, altered, premature junctional beat (PJB)

Atrial-ventricular conduction, altered, Mobitz Type II

Ventricular conduction, altered, premature ventricular beat (PVB)

Serum glucose deficit, hypoglycemia

PANSYSTOLIC/HOLOSYSTOLIC MURMUR

R/O

Alteration in right ventricular-atrial preload

PARALYSIS

R/O
Sexual dysfunction
Intracranial pressure, increased
Cerebral perfusion, obstructed, thromboembolism

PARALYTIC ILEUS

R/O
Intracellular electrolyte deficit, hypokalemia

PARESTHESIA

R/O
Anxiety
Acid–base imbalance, respiratory alkalosis

PERIPHERAL PULSE, DECREASED

R/O
Cardiac output, decreased
Peripheral tissue perfusion, decreased

PINK-TINGED MUCOUS

R/O
Alteration in left ventricular–atrial preload
Extracellular fluid volume excess, alveolar edema

PLEURITIC PAIN

R/O
Pulmonary tissue perfusion, altered, emboli

POLYURIA

R/O
Urinary volume, increased, polyuria
Actual fluid-volume and electrolyte deficit, diabetic shock
Serum glucose excess, hyperglycemia

PULMONARY ARTERY PRESSURE, INCREASED

R/O
    Cardiac output, decreased
    Extracellular fluid volume excess, edema
    Actual whole blood volume deficit, hemorrhagic shock
    Renal tissue perfusion, decreased
    Vasodilatation of vascular bed, septic shock

PULMONARY CAPILLARY WEDGE PRESSURE, DECREASED

R/O
    Intracellular fluid volume deficit, dehydration

PULMONARY CAPILLARY WEDGE PRESSURE, INCREASED

R/O
    Systemic vascular resistance, altered, afterload
    Cardiac output, decreased
    Actual reduction in cardiac output, cardiogenic shock
    Extracellular fluid volume excess, edema
    Actual whole blood volume deficit, hemorrhagic shock
    Renal tissue perfusion, decreased
    Vasodilatation of vascular bed, septic shock

PULSUS ALTERNANS

R/O
    Alteration in left ventricular–atrial preload

PUPILLARY CHANGE

R/O
    Impaired physical mobility, hemiparesis
    Anxiety
    Pain
    Stress
    Arterial blood pressure, altered, hypertension
    Ventricular conduction, altered, ventricular fibrillation

Intracranial pressure, increased
Extracellular fluid volume excess, cerebral edema

RALES/CRACKLES

R/O

Alteration in left ventricular–atrial preload
Cardiac output, decreased
Extracellular volume excess, alveolar edema
Pulmonary tissue perfusion, altered, emboli
Ventilation–perfusion imbalance
Extracellular fluid volume excess, edema
Actual whole blood volume deficit, hemorrhagic shock

REDNESS IN EXTREMITIES

R/O

Peripheral tissue perfusion, obstructed, thromboembolism
Skin integrity, impaired

RIGID BODY LANGUAGE

R/O

Violence directed toward self

SHORTNESS OF BREATH

R/O

Verbal/nonverbal communication deficit
Activity intolerance
Stress
Sinus conduction, altered, sinus tachycardia
Ventricular conduction, altered, ventricular tachycardia
Extracellular fluid volume excess, alveolar edema

S_3

R/O

Alteration in right ventricular–atrial preload
Alteration in left ventricular–atrial preload
Ventricular conduction, altered, ventricular tachycardia
Extracellular fluid volume excess, edema

S$_4$

R/O
   Alteration in right ventricular–atrial preload
   Ventricular conduction, altered, ventricular tachycardia

SEXUAL DRIVE, IMPAIRED

R/O
   Sexual dysfunction

SHORTNESS OF BREATH

R/O
   Verbal/nonverbal communication deficit
   Activity intolerance
   Stress
   Sinus conduction, altered, sinus tachycardia
   Ventricular conduction, altered, ventricular tachycardia
   Extracellular fluid volume excess, alveolar edema

SLOW-HEALING LESIONS

R/O
   Peripheral tissue perfusion, decreased

SPASMS

R/O
   Sexual dysfunction

SPLITTING S$_2$

R/O
   Pulmonary tissue perfusion, altered, emboli

SYNCOPE

R/O
   Alteration in left ventricular–atrial preload
   Cardiac output, decreased
   Sinus conduction, altered, sinus arrhythmia
   Sinus conduction, altered, sinus pause or block

Sinus conduction, altered, SA exit block
Atrial conduction, altered, PAT
Atrial conduction, altered, atrial flutter
Atrial conduction, altered, atrial fibrillation
Atrial–ventricular conduction, altered, junctional tachy-
    cardia
Atrial–ventricular conduction, altered, Mobitz Type I
Atrial–ventricular conduction, altered, complete heart block
Ventricular conduction, altered, ventricular tachycardia

SYSTOLIC BLOOD PRESSURE, INCREASED

R/O
    Intracranial pressure, increased

SYSTEMIC VASCULAR RESISTANCE, INCREASED

R/O
    Cardiac output, decreased

TACHYCARDIA

R/O
    Thought process, altered, confusion
    Verbal/nonverbal communication excess
    Violence directed toward others
    Violence directed toward self
    Activity intolerance
    Loneliness
    Depersonalization
    Anger
    Denial
    Self-concept/self-esteem disturbance
    Body-image disturbance
    Anxiety
    Fear
    Depression
    Loss
    Stress
    Sensory overload

Arterial blood pressure, altered, hypertension
Vasodilatation of vascular bed, anaphylactic shock
Intracranial pressure, increased
Extracellular fluid-volume excess, cerebral edema
Intracellular electrolyte deficit, hypokalemia
Actual fluid-volume and electrolyte deficit, diabetic shock
Intra-abdominal perfusion, decreased
Actual plasma volume deficit, burn shock
Serum glucose excess, hyperglycemia

WEAKNESS

R/O

Activity intolerance
Hopelessness
Anxiety
Pain
Alteration in right ventricular–atrial preload
Systemic vascular resistance, altered, afterload
Cardiac output, decreased
Sinus conduction, altered, sinus bradycardia
Sinus conduction, altered, sinus pause or block
Sinus conduction, altered, SA exit block
Atrial conduction, altered, PAC
Atrial–ventricular conduction, altered, junctional tachy-
cardia
Atrial–ventricular conduction, altered, Mobitz Type I
Atrial–ventricular conduction, altered, Mobitz Type II
Atrial–ventricular conduction, altered, complete heart block
Ventricular conduction, altered, ventricular tachycardia
Cerebral perfusion, obstructed, thromboembolism
Vasodilatation of vascular bed, neurogenic shock
Intracellular fluid volume deficit, dehydration
Extracellular electrolyte excess, hypernatremia
Extracellular electrolyte deficit, hyponatremia
Intracellular electrolyte excess, hypermagnesium
Actual whole blood volume deficit, hemorrhagic shock
Actual whole blood and plasma volume deficit, traumatic
shock
Actual fluid-volume and electrolyte deficit, diabetic shock

Serum glucose excess, hyperglycemia
Serum glucose deficit, hypoglycemia

WEAKNESS ON ONE SIDE

R/O
Impaired physical mobility, hemiparesis
Intracranial pressure, increased
Cerebral tissue perfusion, decreased
Cerebral perfusion, obstructed, thromboembolism

WEIGHT GAIN

R/O
Diversional activity deficit
Cardiac output, decreased
Extracellular fluid volume excess, edema
Extracellular fluid volume excess, intraperitoneal edema or
    ascites

WEIGHT LOSS

R/O
Diversional activity deficit
Psychological immobility
Loneliness
Hopelessness
Self-concept/self-esteem disturbance
Body-image disturbance
Depression
Cardiac output, increased
Intracellular fluid volume deficit, dehydrations
Urinary output, increased, polyuria
Bowel elimination, increased, diarrhea
Nutritional alteration, more than body requirements
Swallowing pattern, altered, dysphagia

WHEEZES

R/O
Alteration in left ventricular–atrial preload

WIDENING PULSE PRESSURE

R/O
    Intracranial pressure, increased
    Extracellular fluid volume excess, cerebral edema

YAWNING

R/O
    Diversional activity deficit

COGNITIVE BEHAVIORS

AGGRESSION

R/O
    Verbal/nonverbal communication excess
    Anger
    Fear

AGITATION

R/O
    Thought process, altered, confusion
    Violence directed toward self
    Family process, altered
    Stress
    Arterial blood pressure, altered, hypotension
    Alteration in distributive gas exchange, spontaneous pneumothorax

ANGER

R/O
    Diversional activity deficit
    Role disturbance
    Family process, altered
    Psychological immobility
    Self-concept/self-esteem disturbance
    Body-image disturbance
    Anxiety

ANXIETY

R/O
   Thought process, altered, confusion
   Verbal/nonverbal communication excess
   Violence directed toward self
   Sexual dysfunction
   Family process, altered
   Impaired physical mobility, hemiparesis
   Activity intolerance
   Loneliness
   Depersonalization
   Powerlessness
   Stress
   Sensory deprivation
   Systemic vascular resistance, altered, afterload
   Cardiac output, decreased
   Coronary artery perfusion, decreased
   Sinus conduction, altered, sinus tachycardia
   Sinus conduction, altered, sinus bradycardia
   Sinus conduction, altered, sinus pause or block
   Sinus conduction, altered, SA exit block
   Atrial conduction, altered, PAT
   Atrial conduction, altered, atrial flutter
   Atrial conduction, altered, atrial fibrillation
   Atrial–ventricular conduction, altered, junctional tachy-
      cardia
   Atrial–ventricular conduction, altered, premature junctional
      beat
   Atrial–ventricular conduction, altered, Mobitz Type I
   Atrial–ventricular conduction, altered, Mobitz Type II
   Atrial–ventricular conduction, altered, complete heart block
   Ventricular conduction, altered, PVB
   Ventricular conduction, altered, ventricular fibrillation
   Ventricular conduction, altered, accelerated idioventricular
      rhythm
   Cardiopulmonary stability, altered, chest injury shock
   Extracellular fluid-volume excess, edema
   Oxygen gas exchange, impaired, alveolar edema
   Acid–base imbalance, respiratory alkalosis

Ineffective breathing pattern, alveolar hypoventilation
Ineffective breathing pattern, alveolar hyperventilation
Ineffective breathing pattern, dyspnea
Pulmonary tissue perfusion, altered, emboli
Ventilation–perfusion imbalance
CNS altered, seizure

APATHY

R/O

Diversional activity deficit
Family process, altered
Psychological immobility
Loneliness
Powerlessness
Self-concept/self-esteem disturbance
Depression
Sensory deprivation
Sleep deprivation
Systemic vascular resistance, altered, afterload
Intracellular electrolyte excess, hyperkalemia

APPREHENSION

R/O

Thought process, altered, confusion
Impaired physical mobility, hemiplegia
Anxiety
Peripheral tissue perfusion, obstructed, thromboembolism
Sinus conduction, altered, sinus pause or block
Sinus conduction, altered, SA exit block
Atrial conduction, altered, PAC
Atrial conduction, altered, PAT
Atrial conduction, altered, atrial flutter
Atrial conduction, altered, atrial fibrillation
Atrial–ventricular conduction, altered, junctional tachy-
cardia
Atrial–ventricular conduction, altered, PJB
Atrial–ventricular conduction, altered, Mobitz Type I
Atrial–ventricular conduction, altered, Mobitz Type II
Atrial–ventricular conduction, altered, complete heart block

Ventricular conduction, altered, PVB
Ventricular conduction, altered, ventricular fibrillation
Ventricular conduction, altered, accelerated idioventricular
    rhythm
Cardiopulmonary stability, altered, chest injury shock
Ineffective breathing pattern, alveolar hypoventilation
Ineffective airway clearance, wheezes
Pulmonary tissue perfusion, altered, emboli
Distributive gas exchange, altered, spontaneous pneumo-
    thorax
Ventilation–perfusion imbalance
CNS altered, seizure
Cerebral perfusion, obstructed, thromboembolism
Vasodilatation of vascular bed, neurogenic shock
Extracellular fluid volume excess, edema
Actual whole blood volume deficit, hemorrhagic shock

ARGUMENTATIVE

R/O
Verbal/nonverbal communication excess
Family process, altered

BELLIGERENCE

R/O
Thought process, altered, confusion

CONFUSION

R/O
Impaired physical mobility, hemiparesis
Impaired physical mobility, hemiplegia
Activity intolerance
Fear
Sensory deprivation
Sleep deprivation
Alteration in left ventricular–atrial preload
Systemic vascular resistance, altered, afterload
Cardiac output, decreased
Arterial blood pressure, altered, hypotension

Psychological immobility
Sleep deprivation
Extracellular fluid volume excess, alveolar edema
Extracellular fluid volume excess, cerebral edema

INABILITY TO SLEEP

R/O
Family process, altered

INAPPROPRIATE SPEECH

R/O
Verbal/nonverbal communication excess

INCOHERENT SPEECH

R/O
Thought process, altered, confusion
Verbal/nonverbal communication excess
Alteration in left ventricular–atrial preload
Speech pattern, altered, aphasia

INSECURITY

R/O
Depersonalization

INTERFERENCE WITH LEARNING

R/O
Hopelessness

IRRITABILITY

R/O
Anxiety
Fear
Depression
Sleep deprivation
Systemic vascular resistance, altered, afterload
Arterial blood pressure, altered, hypertension
Carbon dioxide gas exchange, impaired, hypercapnia

Acid-base imbalance, respiratory alkalosis
Ineffective breathing pattern, alveolar hyperventilation
Ineffective airway clearance, wheezes
Ventilation-perfusion imbalance
Intracranial pressure, increased
Extracellular fluid volume excess, cerebral edema
Cerebral tissue perfusion, decreased
Cerebral tissue obstruction, thromboembolism
Vasodilatation of vascular bed, neurogenic shock
Intracellular electrolyte deficit, hypomagnesium
Urinary output, decreased, oliguria
Urinary output, increased, polyuria
Intra-abdominal perfusion, decreased

LACK OF DECISION MAKING

R/O
Powerlessness
Alteration in left ventricular-atrial preload

LACK OF EYE CONTACT

R/O
Verbal/nonverbal communication deficit
Anger
Self-concept/self-esteem disturbance

LACK OF JUDGMENT

R/O
Oxygen gas exchange, impaired, hypoxemia
Carbon dioxide gas exchange, impaired, hypercapnia

LACK OF KNOWLEDGE

R/O
Role disturbance
Sexual dysfunction
Powerlessness

LACK OF MOTIVATION

R/O
Hopelessness

Anxiety
Depression

LASSITUDE

R/O
Psychological immobility
Sleep deprivation
CNS altered, seizure
Intracellular electrolyte deficit, hypokalemia
Bowel elimination, increased, diarrhea
Vasodilatation of vascular bed, septic shock

LETHARGY

R/O
Systemic vascular resistance, altered, afterload
Arterial blood pressure, altered, hypotension
Extracellular fluid volume excess, alveolar edema
Carbon dioxide gas exchange, impaired, hypercapnia
Acid–base imbalance, respiratory acidosis
Ineffective breathing pattern, alveolar hypoventilation
Ventilation–perfusion imbalance
Intracranial pressure, increased
Extracellular fluid volume excess, cerebral edema
Vasodilatation of vascular bed, neurogenic shock
Extracellular electrolyte excess, hypernatremia
Extracellular electrolyte deficit, hyponatremia
Acid–base imbalance, metabolic acidosis
Extracellular fluid volume excess, intraperitoneal edema or
    ascites
Serum glucose deficit, hypoglycemia

LISTLESSNESS

R/O
Actual fluid volume and electrolyte deficit, diabetic shock

LOOSE ASSOCIATION

R/O
Verbal/nonverbal communication excess

LOSS OF CONTROL

R/O
  Anxiety
  CNS altered, seizure

LOW SELF-ESTEEM

R/O
  Depersonalization

MAGICAL THINKING

R/O
  Denial

MUTENESS

R/O
  Hopelessness

NERVOUSNESS

R/O
  Impaired physical mobility, hemiparesis
  Anxiety
  Arterial blood pressure, altered, hypertension
  Coronary artery perfusion, decreased
  Sinus conduction, altered, sinus bradycardia
  Sinus conduction, altered, sinus pause or block
  Sinus conduction, altered, sinus exit block
  Atrial conduction, altered, PAC
  Atrial conduction, altered, PAT
  Atrial conduction, altered, atrial flutter
  Atrial–ventricular conduction, altered, junctional tachy-
    cardia
  Atrial–ventricular conduction, altered, Mobitz Type I
  Ventricular conduction, altered, PVB
  Alteration in cardiopulmonary stability, chest injury shock
  Acid–base imbalance, respiratory alkalosis
  Ineffective breathing pattern, alveolar hyperventilation
  Ineffective breathing pattern, dyspnea

Vasodilatation of vascular bed, neurogenic shock
Distributive gas exchange, altered, spontaneous pneumothorax

OBSESSIONAL THINKING

R/O
Depersonalization

OBTUNDATION

R/O
Arterial blood pressure, altered, hypotension
Thought process, altered, level of consciousness reduced
Extracellular electrolyte deficit, hyponatremia
Acid–base imbalance, metabolic alkalosis

OVERT AGGRESSIVE ACTS TOWARD OTHERS

R/O
Violence directed toward others

PAIN

R/O
Systemic vascular resistance, altered, afterload
Peripheral tissue perfusion, obstructed, thromboembolism
Sinus conduction, altered, sinus tachycardia
Thought process, altered, level of consciousness reduced
Cerebral tissue perfusion, decreased
Intracellular electrolyte excess, hyperkalemia

PASSIVITY

R/O
Hopelessness

PERCEPTION OF ENVIRONMENT AS THREATENING

R/O
Violence directed toward others

PERCEPTION OF SELF AS WORTHLESS

R/O
    Violence directed toward self

PERSONALIZATION OF INJURED BODY PART

R/O
    Body-image disturbance

PROBLEM SOLVING, DECREASED

R/O
    Family process, altered

PSYCHOTIC THOUGHT PROCESS

R/O
    Violence directed toward self
    Sensory deprivation
    Sleep deprivation
    Oxygen gas exchange, impaired, hypoxemia
    Speech pattern, altered, aphasia

RAPID SPEECH

R/O
    Verbal/nonverbal communication excess

RATIONALIZATION

R/O
    Denial

REDUCED OBJECTIVE THINKING

R/O
    Stress
    Sensory deprivation

REFUSAL TO ACCEPT CHANGE IN SELF

R/O
    Body-image disturbance

REFUSAL TO SPEAK

R/O

Verbal/nonverbal communication deficit

RESIGNATION

R/O

Powerlessness

RESTLESSNESS

R/O

Thought process, altered, confusion
Diversional activity deficit
Impaired physical mobility, hemiplegia
Powerlessness
Self-concept/self-esteem disturbance
Anxiety
Fear
Stress
Sensory deprivation
Sleep deprivation
Cardiac output, decreased
Arterial blood pressure, altered, hypotension
Coronary artery perfusion, decreased
Sinus conduction, altered, sinus tachycardia
Atrial–ventricular conduction, altered, complete heart block
Ventricular conduction, altered, ventricular fibrillation
Extracellular fluid volume excess, alveolar edema
Oxygen gas exchange, impaired, hypoxemia
Acid–base imbalance, respiratory acidosis
Oxygen–carbon dioxide gas exchange imbalance, crackles
Ineffective airway clearance, wheezes
Pulmonary tissue perfusion, altered, emboli
Intracellular fluid volume deficit, dehydration
Extracellular fluid volume excess, edema
Intracellular electrolyte deficit, hypomagnesium
Actual whole blood and plasma volume deficit, traumatic shock
Bowel elimination, uncontrolled, incontinence
Intra-abdominal perfusion, decreased

SARCASM

R/O
  Anger
  Stress

SELECTED PERCEPTION

R/O
  Denial

SELF-CRITICISM

R/O
  Depression

SELF-NEGATING VERBALIZATION

R/O
  Self-concept/self-esteem disturbance
  Depression
  Stress

SILENCE

R/O
  Verbal/nonverbal communication deficit
  Anger
  Speech pattern, altered, aphasia

SLEEP PATTERN, ALTERED

R/O
  Diversional activity deficit
  Family process, altered
  Powerlessness
  Depression
  Carbon dioxide gas exchange, impaired, hypercapnia
  Ineffective breathing pattern, dyspnea
  Intracranial pressure, increased
  Urinary output, increased, polyuria

SUSPICION

R/O
Violence directed toward others

THOUGHT PROCESS, ALTERED

R/O
Coronary artery perfusion, decreased
Extracellular volume excess, edema

THREAT OF PERSONAL LOSS

R/O
Violence directed toward self

TUNNEL VISION

R/O
Denial

UNABLE TO RECOGNIZE OTHERS

R/O
Thought process, altered, confusion

UNREALISTIC EXPECTATION

R/O
Family process, altered

VERBAL ABUSE

R/O
Anger

WEAK OR ABSENT VOICE

R/O
Verbal/nonverbal communication deficit

WITHDRAWAL

R/O
  Thought process, altered, confusion
  Verbal/nonverbal communication deficit
  Noncompliance
  Family process, altered
  Psychological immobility
  Loneliness
  Powerlessness
  Denial
  Self-concept/self-esteem disturbance
  Body-image disturbance
  Anxiety